The Prostate Diet Cookbook

The Prostate Diet Cookbook

Cancer-Fighting Foods for a Healthy Prostate

Buffy Sanders

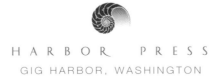

HARBOR PRESS

GIG HARBOR, WASHINGTON

Library of Congress Cataloging-in-Publication Data

Sanders, Buffy.
    The prostate diet cookbook: cancer-fighting foods for a healthy prostate/
Buffy Sanders.
        p. cm.
    Includes bibliographical references and index.
    ISBN 0-936197-42-0 (alk. paper)
        1. Prostate—Diseases—Diet therapy. 2. Prostate—Cancer—Diet therapy.
        I.Title.

RC899 .S26 2001
616.6'50654—dc21

IMPORTANT NOTICE:
The ideas, positions, and statements in this book may in some cases conflict with orthodox mainstream medical opinion, and the advice regarding health matters outlined in this book is not suitable for everyone. Do not attempt self-diagnosis, and do not embark upon self-treatment of any kind without qualified medical supervision. Nothing in this book should be construed as a promise of benefits or of results to be achieved, or a guarantee by the author or publisher of the safety or efficacy of its contents. The author, the publisher, the editor, and its employees disclaim any liability, loss, or risk incurred directly or indirectly as a result of the use or application of any of the contents of this book. If you are not willing to be bound by this disclaimer, please return your copy of the book to the publisher for a full refund.

THE PROSTATE DIET COOKBOOK: Cancer-Fighting Foods for a Healthy Prostate

Printed in the United States of America.
1   3   5   7   9   10   8   6   4   2

Harbor Press, Inc., P.O. Box 1656, Gig Harbor, WA 98335

To Ward Sanders, the love of my life, my joy, my inspiration, my best friend,

and a dedicated husband whose boundless love, unwavering support,

patience, and ongoing encouragement helped make this book a reality.

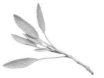

Acknowledgments

▼

This book embodies the ideas, hard work, and generous spirit of many kind people to whom I would like to express my gratitude.

To Kellie Wilson, Judy Kleeves, Judy Knopnicki, Dr. C. Bruce Lee, Dr. Kenneth Peterson, Dr. Celestia Higano, Dr. Michael Brawer, Dorothy Hopper, Marilyn Germano, Laurie Wick, Kathy Bulfin, Patsy Paddison, Toi Woosley, Sawako Sakai, Dr. Hide Sasaki, Marsha Ederer, and Marjorie Wood for their various contributions of recipe ideas, expertise, and moral support; and to members of our prostate cancer support group, Us Too, who encouraged me to write this book and volunteered to test and comment on the recipes.

To Deborah S. Romaine of Textworks for her assistance in bringing the book from draft to final form. To Griggs Irving for finding Harbor Press, just the right publisher. To Alice Colombo for professionally editing the recipes. To Debby Young, Harbor Press editor, for her professionalism, encouragement, and unwavering support of this first-time author.

And my special thanks to Dr. Peter Roffey for his encouragement and enthusiastic support during the writing of this book, and his thorough critique of the completed draft.

Contents

▼

NATURE'S ARSENAL:
Using Nutrition to Fight Prostate Cancer

RECIPES FOR A HEALTHY PROSTATE

Appetizers and Snacks

Beans, Grains, and Vegetable Basics

Soups, Sandwiches, and Salads

Breads and Muffins

Desserts and Treats

Condiments, Sauces, and Spices

Main Dishes

Side Dishes

Foreword

The devastating diagnosis of prostate cancer will be given to approximately 180,000 American men this year. Such a diagnosis has great impact not only on the patient, but also on his family and other loved ones. While we've made strides in our understanding of prostate cancer and in our ability to diagnose and treat it, prostate cancer will be a major health concern for some time to come.

Buffy and Ward Sanders have been battling Ward's prostate cancer for almost a decade. Buffy has truly stood beside Ward and provided stalwart support and a constant source of inspiration. Rather than simply standing by and letting others deal with this difficult situation, Buffy decided to take an active role in helping to manage the disease. She embraced a holistic approach to health, focusing specifically on the effects of nutrition on prostate cancer. The results of this extensive personal study form the basis of this book.

The recipes in *The Prostate Diet Cookbook: Cancer-Fighting Foods for a Healthy Prostate* provide practical approaches for adopting a healthy, low-fat diet, and they incorporate important nutritional recommendations for helping in the battle against prostate cancer. The text accompanying the recipes offers excellent, easy-to-understand guidelines for healthy eating that can be integrated into your lifestyle without difficulty. Because these recipes result in an overall healthier diet, they can be used by everyone—not only people fighting cancer, but also people who have other health problems, or no significant medical conditions at all.

Prostate cancer survivors and their families, as well as those who are trying to prevent prostate cancer, will benefit greatly from the valuable information and recommendations provided here. Just as important, readers will thoroughly enjoy the simple-to-prepare, delicious recipes found throughout this wonderful book!

Michael K. Brawer, M.D.
Director, Northwest Prostate Institute
Seattle, Washington

A Word from Ward

▼

I am the fortunate beneficiary of the work that has gone into this book. During my years of fighting prostate cancer, I have had, with very few exceptions, excellent medical care. At least equally important, I have had the wholehearted, 1000 percent support of Buffy, my partner, friend, lover, and wife. I tell you unequivocally, that without her support, I would be dead now.

To benefit from this book, you must (as I did) change your eating habits. There are tougher things in life. I changed my eating habits when I went from home to college to the Army. I changed once again in early middle age when my metabolism underwent change. And with every change in diet, I found new taste sensations. So it has been with The Prostate Diet. I have discovered a variety of new taste sensations that are helping me to live healthy and live longer — gourmet taste treats from Italy, Japan, China, Thailand, and around the world.

I could do without some of the side effects of prostate cancer, but there have been some positive outcomes as well. I take a little more time to smell the roses. I am more aware of time and the need to use it wisely. My relationship with Buffy is stronger and deeper than ever. And if I hadn't gotten prostate cancer, you wouldn't be reading this book and neither you nor I would be enjoying these gourmet meals. *Bon appétit!*

Ward Sanders

Introduction

▼

One in six men will be diagnosed with prostate cancer during his lifetime. Today in the United States, this means nearly 500 men *each day* find out that they are the "one." Doctors give the life-altering news of prostate cancer to about 180,000 American men every year. And the disease claims the lives of another 40,000 American men each year. All of these figures were just numbers to me until the summer of 1990. That's when my husband Ward—my best friend and the love of my life—became the "one."

Prostate cancer, as those who fight it know all too well, is an unpredictable beast. In some men, it grows so slowly that they will die of other causes long before the prostate cancer even shows signs of its presence. In other men, it sprouts seemingly overnight, invading the body like spring dandelions take over a lawn. And in many men, prostate cancer resides somewhere in-between, sometimes tamed, but always a threat. This middle ground is the turf of Ward's prostate cancer, a battlefield bearing the scars of radiation therapy, cryosurgery, and hormone therapy.

It's hard to sit on the sidelines and watch someone you love fight for his life. Never one for playing the spectator, I wanted to jump in and fight right along with Ward. But what could I do? What I wanted most was to snap my fingers and magically send the cancer away. I've always believed that life is not about sitting around waiting for things to happen, so I turned to my past to help reshape our future.

My degree in psychology had given me strong research skills, so I decided to apply these skills to help Ward. My research took me from medical libraries to my kitchen—and further into my past, to my days growing up on a farm in Michigan. I'd learned to cook with foods fresh from the fields and orchards, vegetables and fruits at their nutritional and flavorful best. I loved nothing more than serving my family steaming carrots, beans, corn, and other vegetables, their brilliant colors as dazzling as the sweet and healthy goodness that crunched from every bite. My passion for good food and gourmet cooking became a way of life.

I already knew that nutrition was important both to maintain health and to recover from illness. But I learned through countless hours of research just how important that connection is. I learned that lifestyle and dietary factors can help cause cancer. I learned that some foods harm and some foods help. I learned that in Japan, where men eat a diet that contains little fat, minimal red meat, and plentiful vegetables, the death rate from prostate cancer is 5.87 per 100,000 compared to 32.19 in the United States. I learned that most doctors, despite their depth of knowledge about medical technology and drugs, are unaware of the large body of research that's been done about the relationship between certain foods and prostate cancer. And I confirmed what I already believed—you can't leave your health (and your life) totally in the hands of modern medicine. It is absolutely essential for you to educate yourself about ways to help your body's natural defenses create an unwelcome, even hostile, environment for cancer.

Encouraged by the many exciting and promising studies of nutrition and prostate cancer, I set out to change our eating habits. I experimented and tested new dishes and revamped old favorites to create a comprehensive, low-fat menu of cancer-fighting meals that are as delicious as they are healthy. Though Ward's cancer still lurks in his body, with the help of good medical care and The Prostate Diet, it has been held at bay for more than ten years. It's the age-old battle tactic of surround and conquer—send as many different weapons as you can to every possible battle line.

While research on the role of diet in the progression of cancer is not yet conclusive, scientists believe that differences in diet and lifestyle play an important part in the wide global variations in the incidence of prostate cancer. We are just beginning to understand how molecules in food and vitamins affect our bodies' cells and energize them to fight cancer. But Ward and I made the decision not to wait for rock-solid scientific proof before changing Ward's diet—and it worked. Ward's prostate-specific antigen, or PSA, level dropped way off, providing a scientific marker that his cancer had indeed retreated.

Our success in "holding the line" against the enemy with the help of my nutrition plan became a topic of conversation at our prostate cancer support group. A member of the group said, "I wish someone would write a cookbook 'just for us men.'" And so I did, and that is how *The Prostate Diet Cookbook* was born.

Research has shown that nearly every man will get prostate cancer if he lives long enough, but by adopting a prostate-healthy diet, you may be able to prevent the cancer from ever becoming a health problem. We know today, more than ever before, that when you switch from a meat-based diet to a plant-based diet, you avoid substances that may help cause cancer, heart disease, and other illnesses, and you consume literally thousands of substances that may protect you against these diseases.

The recipes and nutritional guidelines in this book will help you make an easy transition from your present diet to a menu of foods that will help in your fight against prostate cancer, and promote general good health, as well. I've included quick and easy recipes for every day, extravagant creations that pull out all the stops, elegant dishes, and recipes that are just plain fun. Of course, all of them are simply delicious!

I hope and expect that not only will you benefit from this book, but your entire family will enjoy a healthier, longer life as a result of following the guidelines and using the recipes I have presented here. I wish you success and happy eating!

Nature's Arsenal

Using Nutrition to Fight Prostate Cancer

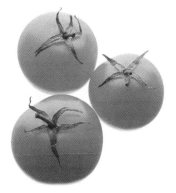

Foods That Fight
Cancer

▼

With a little awareness and planning, you can use foods to give your body the nutrients it needs to help fight — or even help prevent — prostate cancer and sustain your health. The foods you eat provide your body with essential nutrients that your cells use to fuel their functions. Healthy cells crave vitamins, minerals, trace elements, and antioxidants to keep them strong and resistant to being taken over by cancer cells. These substances are abundant in vegetables, fruits, whole grains, soybeans, and legumes. Cancer cells, particularly those of hormone-driven cancers such as prostate cancer, seem to thrive on other substances such as alpha-linolenic acid, arachidonic acid, and other fatty acids. These are abundant in foods that come from animal sources including meat, egg yolks, and milk and other dairy products.

Most of the foods that help fight prostate cancer contain combinations of cancer-fighting substances. Researchers don't fully understand whether it is the individual substances or the collaboration that makes such foods effective. Sometimes scientists aren't able to demonstrate in the laboratory how a particular food works to combat prostate cancer, yet the evidence that it does seems apparent when looking at real people — what researchers call anecdotal evidence.

For example, Japan, where people eat mostly vegetables and soy products, has one of the world's lowest prostate cancer death rates. The United States, on the other hand, where the basic diet is meat, dairy, and potatoes, has one of the highest death rates from prostate cancer in the world. Japanese men who eat a traditional Japanese diet consume five times the amount of cancer-fighting substances as their American counterparts. Further, studies show that in men who emigrate from Japan to the United States the death rate from prostate cancer climbs in proportion to the length of time they live in this country. This points a steady finger at the role of vegetables and soy products in preventing, or at least reducing the spread of, prostate cancer.

Nature's Four Warriors Against Prostate Cancer

The key food-related warriors in the battle against prostate cancer appear to be four camps of chemical substances — isoflavones, sulforaphanes, lycopenes, and polyphenols.

■ **Isoflavones** appear in the highest concentrations in soybeans. One of the most important isoflavones is genistein. Genistein appears to inhibit the growth of prostate cancer cells, keeping them from spreading to other parts of the body. Soy foods that contain isoflavones include tofu, tempeh, miso, and soy protein isolate. Cooking does not seem to alter the concentration or effectiveness of soy's isoflavones, though processed soy products such as soy burgers have lower concentrations.

■ **Sulforaphanes** are the primary cancer-fighting chemicals in cruciferous vegetables such as broccoli, cabbage, kale, and cauliflower. You receive the most nutritional value from these vegetables when you eat them raw or lightly cooked.

■ **Lycopenes** are found primarily in tomatoes. You receive the highest level of lycopenes from cooked tomatoes and food products such as tomato paste, sauce, and juice. Heat during cooking changes the chemical formulation of lycopene into one more easily digested by the human body. Watermelon and pink grapefruit also contain lycopenes, though in much lower concentrations than tomatoes.

Polyphenols are found in green tea. The most potent polyphenol in the war against prostate cancer is called epigallocatechin gallate, or EGCG. In laboratory tests on mice, EGCG significantly slows the growth of new blood vessels, cutting off the supply of nutrients to cancer tumors. EGCG also appears to prevent cancer cells from dividing, which stops their growth.

Like any well-directed army, these four warriors battle prostate cancer on different fronts. A daily diet that includes foods to provide all of them helps fortify your body's natural defenses.

These data from the Journal of the National Cancer Institute show the death rate from prostate cancer in various countries where the average life expectancy of men is over 70 years:

Country	Prostate Cancer Deaths (men out of every 100,000)	Average Life Expectancy (only countries higher than 70)
New Zealand	35.09	73
Uruguay	34.94	73
Belgium	33.78	73
Germany	32.21	73
United States	32.19	75
France	31.43	75
Austria	31.23	74
The Netherlands	29.98	76
Cuba	29.86	75
Canada	29.20	73
England	28.38	74
Scotland	27.40	74
Italy	22.57	74
Greece	15.83	74
Singapore	7.47	72
Japan	5.87	77
Hong Kong	5.44	75

While the life expectancy is nearly equal in these countries, the prostate cancer death rates are significantly different. Researchers believe that the wide global variations in the incidence of prostate cancer are in part explained by differences in diet and lifestyle. Note that the incidence rates in Singapore, Japan, and Hong Kong are 1/5 or less than that of the U.S. (and other countries with similar diet and lifestyle) due to, we believe, the low-fat, high-soy, and vegetable-rich diet in these countries.

The Prostate

Diet

By following The Prostate Diet, you will be able to avoid foods that help to cause prostate cancer while at the same time providing nourishment to other cells in your body that help fight cancer and that keep the rest of your body healthy. The more we learn about nutrition, the more we recognize the truth in the adage "you are what you eat." Every day your body needs certain foods and the nutrients they provide to repair and replace damaged cells, manufacture hormones and enzymes, and maintain the chemical balance that is necessary for good health.

These simple nutritional guidelines will help you choose foods that help fight prostate cancer and avoid foods that promote the growth of prostate cancer cells:

- Get the fat out of your diet.

- Eliminate meat and dairy products.

- Load up on soy protein.

- Eat lots of vegetables, especially cruciferous and tomatoes.

- Drink green tea.

Get the Fat Out of Your Diet

One goal of The Prostate Diet is to keep overall fat intake at 10 to 15 percent, which is well below the average American's level of nearly 40 percent. Cutting meat and dairy products from your diet will make a substantial difference. But even on a plant-based diet, you still have to be careful. Fat can lurk where you least expect to find it. Soybeans, for example, are high in fat, but if you are careful about your overall fat intake, the benefits you will get from soybeans will far outweigh the risks.

Foods That Fight Prostate Cancer

Many foods appear to contain substances (isoflavones) that stop the growth of, and sometimes even kill, prostate cancer cells. Foods that help fight prostate cancer include:

- Soybeans

- Soy products such as tofu, tempeh, soymilk, soy flour, and textured vegetable protein (TVP)

- Cruciferous vegetables such as cabbage, broccoli, kale, and cauliflower

- Tomatoes, particularly cooked

- Red-fleshed fruits such as pink grapefruit, guava, and watermelon

- Green tea

These foods also provide other vital nutrients to bolster your immune system and improve your body's ability to fight disease in general.

■ ■ ■ ■ ■ ■ ■ ■ ■

Foods That Fuel Prostate Cancer Growth

Some foods appear to spur the growth of prostate cancer cells. These are most often foods, such as animal fats, that contain arachidonic acids. These foods encourage your body to produce more testosterone, which feeds prostate cancer cells. Foods to avoid include:

- Meat

- Dairy products containing fat

- Egg yolks (egg whites are OK)

Eliminating these foods from your diet reduces the challenges your body faces, allowing your natural defenses to focus their efforts on fighting your prostate cancer.

Some of the recipes in this book that feature soybeans and soy products may contain more than 15 percent fat in order to provide a rich source of isoflavones and other nutrients. For most men, this is an acceptable trade-off as long as the average fat intake in a week is within the 15 percent limit. Plan your menus over the week instead of day-to-day, and add extra servings of vegetables, especially cruciferous, to boost your intake of other cancer-fighting substances.

Beware Added Fat

A diet based on vegetables and grains is naturally low in saturated and polyunsaturated fats. Yet adding just one teaspoon of oil for cooking can add five grams of fat to your food, or 45 calories. If the food contains 100 calories to start with, this one teaspoon of oil raises its fat content to 45 percent!

Processed convenience foods also contain high quantities of fat. While canned beans or tomatoes are often easier to use (and some of the recipes in this book call for them), it can be just as easy to make your own in double batches and freeze half for later use. If you buy processed foods, read the labels carefully and buy those that are fat-free or, if the product contains oil, make sure it's olive oil.

Olive Oil: The "Good" Fat

Sometimes you need to use a little oil for sautéing and cooking. In such circumstances, use olive oil or olive oil spray. However, olive oil does contain fat, so you still have to use it sparingly. And excess fat in your diet becomes excess fat in your body. This encourages increased testosterone production, which fuels prostate cancer cells (see page 14). Measure the olive oil that you use, so you know how much fat you're adding to your food.

Low-Fat Cooking Options

Baking, broiling, blanching, microwaving, steaming, and sautéing with liquids are popular

Replace Meat with Soy

Cutting down on fat is essential ... but not enough. Soy protein contains a nutrient called genistein that appears to fight all hormone-driven cancers, including prostate cancer. Whenever possible, substitute tofu or tempeh for meat in your favorite recipes. These foods are especially high in soy protein and genistein, and can add both flavor and texture to the dishes you prepare.

ways to cook foods without added oils and fats. These preparation methods showcase the natural flavors of the foods. Start with the freshest foods possible for the fullest flavor and texture. Try these cooking methods to add flavor and cut fat:

- **Baking** – Uses the oven to cook foods. Baked vegetables can serve as side dishes or can be used in other dishes to enhance the depth of flavor.

- **Broiling** – Cooks foods briefly with high heat.

- **Blanching** – Plunges vegetables briefly into boiling water to soften them slightly, then dips them into cold water to stop the cooking process. The result is vegetables that are still somewhat crisp. Blanching also intensifies the color of green vegetables.

- **Microwaving** – Cooks foods from the inside out, quickly and without destroying vital nutrients.

- **Steaming** – Cooks foods in a tightly-covered pot over a small amount of boiling water.

- **Sautéing or stir-frying with liquids** – Uses hot liquids to quickly cook foods in a skillet or wok. Conventional sautéing, or stir-frying, uses a small amount of cooking oil, but the recipes in this book use liquids such as vegetable broth or cooking sherry to give foods a deep, rich flavor.

If you stir-fry the conventional way, use a small amount of olive oil spray in a hot wok or skillet. Don't overcook. This is a common mistake that can drain the flavor and nutrients from foods, especially vegetables. Combine vegetable dishes with an eye to complementary colors, flavors, and textures. When serving cooked vegetables, a crisp green salad is a great companion.

Foods that Help Remove Fats from the Body

Not all fats are bad for you, of course. Indeed, your body requires certain fats for cell repair and function. Eliminating meat and dairy products from your diet still leaves you with other sources for the fats your body needs. Eat more whole grains and fiber-rich vegetables and fruits to help move excess fat through your body. This allows your body to extract what it needs without storing extra dietary fat in the form of fatty acids.

▼ Eliminate Meat and Dairy

Thanks to much media coverage and extensive efforts to spread the word about the role of fat in heart disease, most Americans are at least aware that a diet high in fat, especially saturated or animal fat, is not healthy for anyone. What many are surprised to learn, however, is that the fats found primarily in meat and dairy products that are blamed for clogged arteries also appear to be responsible for speeding the growth of a number of cancers. This correlation is strongest for hormone-driven cancers such as prostate cancer.

The Testosterone Connection

Testosterone is the primary male hormone. Produced by the testicles, and, in lesser quantities, by the adrenal glands, testosterone gives a man's body its male characteristics. Unfortunately, this hormone also becomes a fuel line for prostate cancer cells.

Prostate cancer treatment usually targets two goals: the cancerous tumor itself (through surgery, radiation, or chemotherapy) and its fuel supply (through hormone suppression therapy). Saturated fats such as those found in meats and dairy products convert into substances in your body that increase testosterone production. Excess body fat also provides a steady source of these same substances.

Experts recommend maintaining an appropriate body weight and eliminating meat and dairy products from your diet to help shut down this conversion process.

All health experts recommend a diet low in saturated fats as a pathway to optimal health. Many who specialize in treating prostate cancer take this recommendation a step further, encouraging a vegetarian or vegan (no animal products at all) diet. A diet high in animal fat appears to increase the body's testosterone production. This has the same effect on prostate cancer cells that high-octane gasoline has on your car — increased acceleration.

The correlation is strongest in the presence of two fatty acids, alpha-linolenic acid and arachidonic acid, which make prostate cancer cells thrive and reproduce at a greater rate. Your body produces these substances when it metabolizes meats, dairy products, egg yolks, polyunsaturated cooking oils, margarine, and mayonnaise containing fat. Scientists call these foods precursors — they produce these hazardous fatty acids. However, olive oil appears to be a neutral oil that you can use sparingly. The Prostate Diet should eliminate as many precursor foods as possible. This has the added advantage of reducing your overall fat intake, which ideally should be no more than 15 percent of your calories.

Legumes can help fill in the protein gap left by eliminating meat from your diet. In addition to being a good source of protein, legumes — beans, peas, adzuki, lentils, chickpeas — also provide vitamins (especially B vitamins), minerals such as calcium and iron, and fiber. Legumes are low in calories and fat, and contain no saturated fat or cholesterol. They can also lower testosterone levels. Soybeans are the only legumes that contain isoflavones, however.

Soy products are popular meat substitutes. Foods such as tofu, tempeh, and textured vegetable protein (TVP) can provide texture and flavor to many dishes that traditionally use meat, such as chili and casseroles (see page 17). Many soy-based foods are also high in prostate cancer-fighting isoflavones, especially genistein.

The Poultry Debate

Meats are among the foods that produce a fatty acid called arachidonic acid, which is believed to provide fuel for prostate cancer cells. Red meats produce the highest levels of archidonic acid, while poultry (chicken and turkey) produce low levels.

For many years, prostate cancer experts believed that the level of archidonic acid in poultry was so low that a moderate amount of skinless chicken and turkey breast was not harmful to men with prostate cancer. Now, however, some experts believe that any amount of archidonic acid is harmful, and they recommend a strict vegan (plant-based) diet for men with prostate cancer.

Research findings are not yet conclusive, and studies on the link between archidonic acid and prostate cancer continue.

Milk and other dairy products aren't good for you when you're fighting prostate cancer. Some studies suggest that drinking just two glasses of whole milk a day can raise a man's risk for prostate cancer by 40 percent. The culprit seems to be the fat found in dairy products. Fatty dairy products, therefore, are off limits for prostate cancer survivors and for men who want to significantly lower their risk for prostate cancer. Fortunately, it's easy to eliminate dairy from your diet and still eat nutritious, balanced meals.

Nondairy Milks

There are many varieties of nondairy milks available in most grocery stores. Soymilks are the most popular, though there are also milks made from rice. Nondairy milks are ideal for cooking and work well in just about any recipe that calls for milk, including puddings, cakes, cream sauces, and soups. They are also good over breakfast cereal.

Is It Dairy … or Is It Tofu?

Tofu is a great dairy substitute, both because it contains prostate-cancer fighting isoflavones and because it lacks the fats and arachidonic acids found in cream and cheese (see page 14). Soft tofu, blended and flavored with salt and fresh parsley, is a perfect replacement for ricotta cheese in stuffing pasta shells or making lasagna. Tofu is also great as a substitute for sour cream (blend with fresh lemon juice) or whipped cream (whip with sugar and a dash of lemon). Blend tofu into dishes that call for cream, and mix tofu with herbs and lemon juice to create a tasty spread.

Load Up on Soy Protein

Soybeans contain high amounts of substances called protease inhibitors, which block or slow cancer cell growth especially in hormone-driven cancers such as prostate cancer. Soybeans also contain isoflavones, including genistein, phytosterols, phytoestrogens, and saponins — all chemical substances known to interfere with the growth of cancer cells. Some studies suggest saponins also stimulate the immune system, improving its ability to kill and repel cancer cells.

Vitamin D from the Sun

Studies show that vitamin D, which most people get primarily from sunlight and dairy products, helps reduce the growth of prostate cancer. There is a higher incidence of hormone-related cancers in northern Europe and the northern United States, where there is less sunlight, than in the southern parts of these countries. To help replace the vitamin D you might otherwise get from dairy products, get more sun! Limit your exposure, of course, to prevent sunburn. About fifteen minutes a day will do it. (If you're going to be in the sun for longer than fifteen minutes a day, be sure to use sunscreen.)

Foods from Soy

Though soybeans are a great source of cancer-fighting substances as well as protein, their tough outer skins and dense inner cores make them a challenge for the human digestive system. Most people can tolerate eating only small quantities of the beans directly. Soy products are a common and tasty substitute for straight soybeans. Some processed soy products made with soy protein concentrate, such as soy burgers, may not contain very high concentrations of isoflavones, depending on the processing methods used. Here are some popular and easy-to-find soy products:

- **Miso.** This condiment comes in the form of a smooth paste. It adds flavor to soups, dressings, and marinades, and is particularly popular in Japanese cooking.

- **Soy cheese.** Made from soymilk, soy cheese has a somewhat creamy texture. You can use it as a substitute for cream cheese or to top pizza.

- **Soy flour.** Ground from roasted soybeans, soy flour comes in three varieties. Natural soy flour contains the oils from the soybeans. Defatted soy flour has the oils removed. Lecithinated soy flour has lecithin added, an emulsifying agent that improves stability and reduces crystallization. You can use soy flour as you would use wheat flour.

- **Soy protein isolate powder.** Available in health food markets, soy protein isolate powder is drawn from defatted soy flakes. At more than 90 percent protein, soy protein isolate is one of the most concentrated forms of protein available. It's easily digestible and can be added to many dishes without altering their flavor or texture.

- **Soymilk.** The fluid that results when soybeans are soaked, then ground and strained, is called soymilk. Some soymilk is fortified with calcium and vitamin D. You can use soymilk in any way you would use cow's milk, including to drink straight, pour over cereal, and mix into recipes.

- **Soy yogurt.** Made from soymilk, soy yogurt is very similar to dairy yogurt in consistency. Many health food stores sell flavored soy yogurt.

- **Tempeh.** Made from fermented soybeans and sometimes other grains, tempeh is chunky and tender with a somewhat nutty flavor. Tempeh is a good meat substitute in heartier dishes such as casseroles, soups, and chili.

- **Textured vegetable protein (TVP).** TVP offers a meat-like taste and texture that's easy on the digestive system and high in protein. TVP products are often shaped, colored, and flavored to mimic meat products such as hotdogs, hamburgers, bacon, Canadian bacon, and pepperoni.

- **Tofu.** Also called soybean curd, tofu has little flavor by itself and comes in different textures. Tofu is rich in protein and B vitamins, and comes in soft, medium, and firm textures. Firm tofu is easy to cut or cube and is an ideal meat substitute, or can be chunked to replace ricotta cheese in recipes. Soft tofu has a texture similar to cream cheese and works well as a substitute for cream cheese or sour cream in recipes. Silken tofu is creamy and works well in sauces, dips, and dressings.

- **Yuba.** When hot soymilk cools, a skin forms on the top. Peeled and dried, this skin becomes yuba, a popular ingredient in many Asian recipes.

Getting Your Daily Genistein

You can get the recommended 30 to 50 milligrams a day of genistein from:

- ½ cup tempeh (60 mg.)

- 1 to 3 cups of soymilk (20 mg. per cup)

- 1 to 2 cups of tofu (38 mg. per cup)

- ½ cup roasted soybeans (80 mg.)

- ½ cup cooked green soybeans (70 mg.)

Genistein is also available as a supplement that you can buy at most health food stores and many grocery stores.

▼ Eat Your Vegetables

Your mother had it right when she said, "Eat your vegetables!" Scientists are now verifying the value of this ageless advice. Vegetables are emerging as a leading factor in maintaining health, as well as in fighting disease. A recent study in the Journal of the National Cancer Institute reports that men who eat three or more servings of vegetables a day decrease their risk for developing prostate cancer by 48 percent. Men who eat even more servings daily further decrease their risk.

Fresh is best, since vegetables (and fruits) begin losing nutrients as soon as they are picked, so get as close to the source as possible. Many people enjoy cultivating gardens to grow the fruits and vegetables they enjoy. Health food markets and specialty grocery stores also offer a good variety of fresh produce. When you do cook vegetables, use methods that preserve as many nutrients as possible, such as blanching and steaming (see page 13).

Thanks to rapid transportation and modern refrigeration methods, it's possible to get fresh vegetables year-round in most locations. If you can't always get your vegetables fresh, you can substitute frozen vegetables. Though processing siphons some of their nutritional value, frozen vegetables still provide good levels of vitamins, minerals, and other nutrients. Frozen vegetables are especially handy for adding flavor, variety, and color to your favorite dishes.

Avoid canned vegetables. The processing that canned vegetables are subjected to robs them of nearly all of their nutrients. The one exception is tomatoes. The high temperatures used in processing convert lycopenes in tomatoes into a form that makes these prostate cancer-fighting substances easier for your body to absorb and use (see page 21).

At the Head of the Line: Cruciferous Vegetables

"Cruciferous" isn't a word you would instinctively associate with good health, or even something you would want to put in your mouth. But the vegetables that fall under this cumbersome moniker are among the most powerful weapons in nature's arsenal of disease-fighting foods. The most familiar of these include broccoli, cauliflower, Brussels sprouts, kale, and cabbage. Recently scientists have determined that cruciferous vegetables contain sulforaphane, a chemical substance that increases the activities of prostate cancer-fighting enzymes in your body. Three-day-old sprouts from broccoli seeds contain 30 to 50 times the amount of sulforaphane than mature broccoli. You can buy broccoli seeds in health food stores and sprout your own. Researchers at the Fred Hutchinson Cancer Research Center report that just three servings a week of cruciferous vegetables can reduce by 41 percent a man's risk of developing prostate cancer.

Think Red for Prostate Health: Tomatoes

A number of studies link eating tomatoes and tomato products with a lower risk for prostate cancer. Experts believe this has to do with chemical substances called lycopenes, which occur in high concentrations in tomatoes. Cooked tomatoes and products made with cooked tomatoes have the highest levels of lycopenes. The high temperatures of cooking changes the chemical form of the lycopenes into a formulation your body can more readily use. Olive oil gives lycopenes even more power. One serving of dried tomatoes packed in olive oil delivers sixteen times the amount of lycopenes as a raw tomato (be sure to drain off the excess oil). Cooking tomatoes in a small amount of olive oil also increases the amount of lycopene your body can absorb.

Beyond Broccoli – Cruciferous Vegetables

Adding more cruciferous vegetables can be an adventure in colors, flavors, and textures. The cruciferous vegetable family includes:

Arugula	Horseradish
Beet greens	Kale
Bok choy	Kohlrabi
Broccoli	Mustard greens
Brussels sprouts	Radishes
Cabbage	Rutabaga
Cauliflower	Swiss chard
Chinese cabbage	Turnips and turnip greens
Collard greens	Watercress
Daikon	

If you cook your cruciferous vegetables, use methods such as steaming, blanching, or microwaving to preserve nutrients (see page 13).

Drink Green Tea

Green tea is emerging as a leading natural cancer-fighter. Once viewed as nothing more than wishful thinking, green tea is now commanding the attention of researchers worldwide. Green tea contains high levels of a group of chemical substances called polyphenols. These chemicals appear capable of a wide range of healing functions, from diminishing damage from sun exposure to interfering with the actions of cancer-causing substances. In research studies, polyphenols — in particular, one called epigallocatechin gallate or EGCG — have been found to cause cancer cells to stop growing in cancers involving the prostate gland, as well as in other parts of the body, such as the breast, lungs, and colon.

EGCG seems to attack in a multi-pronged way. On one level of attack, it interferes with the body's process of developing new blood vessels, called angiogenesis. This prevents cancerous tumors from getting to the blood supply, and thus the nutrients, that they need

Lycopene Content Guide

Cooked tomato products provide the highest levels of lycopenes. Here is the lycopene content of some popular foods in milligrams per serving (about 3½ ounces, or 100 grams, which is slightly less than ½ cup).

Food	Amount of Lycopene in Milligrams
Tomato powder	100-125
Dried tomato in oil	50
Canned pizza sauce	13
Catsup	10-13
Tomato soup	8
Tomato sauce	6
Tomato juice	5-12
Fresh guava	5
Cooked tomatoes	4
Raw pink grapefruit	3
Fresh watermelon	2-7
Fresh papaya	2-5

to survive and grow. On a second level of attack, EGCG interferes with the cell division process by which prostate cancer cells reproduce. This slows the tumor's growth. Some studies suggest that in very high doses (the equivalent of ten cups of green tea daily), EGCG causes existing prostate cancer cells to die.

Choose brands of green tea that are pure green tea, whenever possible. Some brands blend green tea with other kinds of tea. The higher the percentage of green tea, the greater the amount of cancer-fighting EGCG. Serve green tea at the end of a meal, for a teatime break, or iced with lemon and mint. You can also add green tea powder, which is available in capsule form at many health food stores, to smoothies and other drinks. Green tea extracts are usually far more concentrated than the tea itself and they are often decaffeinated, making it easier to take high doses.

Eat Plenty of Fruits for Good Health

Fruits are high in antioxidants, chemical substances that help your body get rid of the natural toxins of cell activity called free radicals. In high concentrations, free radicals kill healthy cells outright. In low concentrations, free radicals damage DNA, the cell's genetic material.

Many experts believe this damage sets the stage for cancer to invade the cells. Antioxidants neutralize free radicals, preventing them from doing damage.

As with vegetables, fruits are most nutritious when they're fresh. Citrus fruits offer the highest levels of cancer-fighting substances for cancers in general.

Eat a Wide Variety
of Nutritious Foods

▼

In general, a balanced and nutritious diet helps your body stay healthy and fight disease. Eating a wide variety of foods from the different food groups gives you a broad spectrum of vitamins, minerals, and other vital nutrients. Fruits, vegetables, and whole grains are rich sources of dietary fiber as well, which is important for general good health. Fiber is especially important in the fight against prostate cancer because it absorbs dietary fat before your digestive system has a chance to break down fats into the fatty acids that fuel the growth of prostate cancer cells.

▼ Variety and Portions

It's easy to create meals that are as delicious as they are good for you. The recipes in this book offer a great start as you make changes in your eating habits. You can virtually travel the world without leaving your kitchen by preparing dishes from various countries. Plan your meals a week at a time to give yourself variety and balanced nutrition. If you're fighting prostate cancer now and your appetite varies, eat nutrient-packed foods when you're feeling better to make up for the times when you feel less well. And if you're suffering from nausea or loss of appetite, try frequent but smaller meals.

Traditionally, Americans tend to think of main dishes and side dishes in terms of portion sizes. The main dish is the largest serving, while side dishes are smaller servings. The Prostate Diet looks instead at variety. What matters most is getting enough servings of vegetables, fruits, soy products, whole grains (which are generally more nutritious than processed grains), and legumes. Servings are generally of equal size, with vegetables dominating the meal.

Portion control is important with legumes (including soybeans), grains, and carbohydrates (pasta, rice, breads). In large quantities, legumes can create problems for your digestive system, such as gas and bloating. Your body converts excess amounts of grains and carbohydrates into fat, which then becomes a fuel supply for prostate cancer cells. You can eat as much as you want (and more) of most vegetables and fruits. Instead of one side dish of vegetables, have two or more, both cooked and raw. But don't eat that big platter of pasta and only a tiny serving of vegetables.

Portion Guide

- Limit dietary fat to no more than 15% of your total calories per day.

- Consume 30 to 50 grams of soy protein each day.

- Consume 25 to 35 grams of dietary fiber each day.

- Eat four to seven servings of vegetables each day.

- Eat two to four servings of fruit each day.

What About Sugar
and Salt?

▼

There is no direct correlation between either sugar or salt and prostate cancer. However, a diet high in either (or both) is not good for your health in general, and, indirectly, may have an impact on prostate cancer. A healthful diet — which, among other things, is low in sugar and low in salt — helps your body maintain a strong immune system, giving you the best possible defense against health challenges ranging from colds and viral infections to prostate cancer. In addition, your body converts extra sugar into body fat, which puts you at a higher risk for prostate cancer (see page 10).

Both sugar and salt can "hide" in processed foods, taking on different forms that are nonetheless still sugar and salt. Sugar might appear as fructose or sucrose, for example, which are forms typically found in fruits and naturally sweet substances such as honey. These sugars are also used as sweeteners in a wide variety of food products including items you might not think of as sweet, such as prepared spaghetti sauce. Salt is known chemically as sodium chloride, and is used in many chemical compounds because of its preservative effects. (The earliest form of preserving foods such as meat was to soak them in brine, a salt water solution.) Salt is also the world's most popular seasoning.

Most people consume far more sugar and salt in their diets than they realize. Even when you're being careful, it's easy to overdo it. The forms and amounts of sugar and salt that occur naturally in fruits and vegetables are not nearly as troublesome as those that are present in prepared or processed foods. You need some sugar and salt in your diet, of course, but experts generally recommend limiting the salt and sugar you consume.

Nutrition and Benign Prostate
Hyperplasia (BPH)

▼

The Prostate Diet may be beneficial not only for men who are concerned about prostate cancer, but also for men who are concerned about other common prostate conditions, such as benign prostate hyperplasia (BPH). BPH, which affects 1 out of 3 men over the age of 50, and 8 out of 10 men 80 years old and over, is a noncancerous prostate condition characterized by abnormal enlargement of the prostate.

While there have been literally thousands of research studies linking nutrition with prostate cancer, unfortunately, there has been little research done on the relationship between nutrition and other prostate conditions such as BPH. The research that is available, however, suggests an increased incidence of BPH in men whose diets are high in fat and animal protein, and low in vegetables and whole grains. If you follow the guidelines in The Prostate Diet, which is low in fat and rich in vegetables, you'll be ahead of the game in insuring your overall prostate health, and your general good health as well.

Supplementing Mother Nature
Vitamins and Minerals

▼

Your body's cells need vitamins and minerals, among other substances, to fuel their daily functions. Most experts believe that a healthy adult should be able to meet his or her body's nutritional needs by eating a balanced diet and getting regular exercise (exercise helps the body more efficiently use many substances). Giving your body's cells more than what they need does not seem to improve their functions. With fat-soluble vitamins (vitamins A, D, E, and K) and most minerals, taking too much can lead to serious and even fatal health problems.

BUT (and this is an important qualifier) when your body is fighting disease, it drains its resources much more quickly. Treatments such as chemotherapy, radiation therapy, and surgery also drain your body's nutritional and immune resources. Replenishing vital vitamins and minerals can help your body recharge more quickly, bolstering your immune system so it can carry on a strong defense against invading cancer cells and other challenges.

Health experts recommend these nutritional supplements to help fight prostate cancer:

- **Selenium** 200 mcg/day

- **Vitamin E** 50 IU/day

- **Zinc** 50 mg. two times a day

It's important to maintain a nutritional balance that supports your body's health. Be sure to talk with your doctor before you start a diet high in particular nutrients or start taking any supplements. Some substances can interfere with certain medical treatments or must be taken with caution.

The Importance of Regular
Exercise

▼

Regular exercise is, of course, a staple of good health. It keeps your bones strong, muscles toned, and cardiovascular system (heart, lungs, and circulation) in peak operating condition. One inescapable inevitability of growing older is that body systems begin to weaken and wear out. When you're 70, your balance isn't what it was when you were 50 … or 30. Regular exercise can postpone and even reduce deterioration in nearly everyone, improving health and your sense of well-being.

When you have prostate cancer, however, regular exercise becomes more than a fountain of youth. Exercise helps your body combat the effects of hormone therapy, one of the treatment options for prostate cancer. Hormone therapy suppresses testosterone, a hormone that is largely responsible for giving a man's body its muscle structure and mass. When testosterone levels become low as a result of the hormone therapy, your body loses muscle mass, tone, and strength, and fat replaces the lost muscle tissue. Exercise helps fight this accumuation of body fat and builds muscle tone. Specific exercises that target certain areas of the body help you maintain muscle strength and overall flexibility.

And let's not overlook exercise's role in helping you *feel* better. It's not just that exercise increases your metabolism, speeding the removal of natural toxins from your body to make way for additional nutrients. Exercise, especially strenuous activity such as fast walking or jogging, also releases natural chemicals in your body that send signals of pleasure to your brain. This relieves stress and calms you. These "feel good" messages give you a natural high, setting the stage for a good mood that can last for hours after the exercise stops.

One of the easiest forms of exercise for most people is walking. It requires no special equipment (though good walking shoes are a smart investment), and you can do it outside or indoors (many shopping malls open early to accommodate walkers). If regular exercise is new to you, start slowly. Walk for 15 minutes every other day until this feels comfortable. Take the stairs instead of the elevator (rest if you need to), and park at the back of the parking lot so you can walk to the office or store entrance. Gradually increase both the length and intensity of your walks, until you're walking 45 minutes a day five days a week. Let your interests guide you in other activities. Gardening and yard work offer a surprising workout. Many people also enjoy golf, tennis, bowling, sailing, bicycling, and other strenuous or competitive sports.

Discuss your exercise plans with your doctor, especially if it's been a while since you've done anything more active than reach for the TV remote. As good for you as exercise is, it also requires resources from your body. You might need to build up to the level of exercise your body can support.

Activities that Exercise Your Body

Many of your favorite activities can also provide the regular exercise your body needs to stay healthy and keep your prostate cancer at bay.

- Take a vigorous walk at lunchtime. Walk around the block, to the post office, to the store.

- Play a round of golf and walk the holes.

- Give away the bread-making machine. Kneading dough is probably one of the most soul-satisfying activities ever invented.

- For long telephone calls, use a cordless phone so you can walk upstairs, downstairs, and even around the garden or yard.

- Lift cans of tomatoes or sacks of dried beans one at a time to their places in the cupboard (and call it domestic weight training!).

When physical activity becomes a regular part of your daily routine, your body functions more efficiently. This improves its ability to maintain your good health.

Nurture Your Spirit,
Strengthen Your Body

▼

Your body is an amazing system. The cells and tissues you ordinarily think about in connection to health and disease are really elements of an intricate and complex network. Though you focus on certain organs and structures when you're fighting disease or illness, your whole being becomes involved in the battle. Extending beyond physical boundaries to play a critical role in your response and your recovery are your emotions and your spirit. Your ability to maintain a positive attitude and to deal with the stresses of a serious medical challenge like prostate cancer can have as much of an effect on your well-being as any medical treatment.

Doctors have hundreds of stories about people who beat seemingly unbeatable odds through their faith and determination that they would prevail. "Such a positive attitude. Such a strong spirit!" they say in a tone that blends awe and disbelief. Doctors also have countless stories about people who could do well but instead give up, cutting their lives short. As you embark on what could be the most significant battle of your life, this fight against prostate cancer, it's as important to nurture your spirit as to nourish your body. Meditate, pray, contemplate — whatever it is that helps you reach beyond yourself for strength and comfort. Enlist the support of family and friends to share your successes and lift you up when you're feeling low.

Tips for Delicious and
Easy-to-Prepare Dishes

▼

The recipes in this book are delicious, as well as healthy and easy to prepare. You can buy most ingredients at major grocery stores. Other ingredients might require a trip to a health food market or purchasing through mail order sources.

Adding Flavor to Foods with Herbs and Spices

Herbs and spices offer a great way to vary the flavor of your favorite foods. Some may also have anti-cancer properties. Curcumin, which is often used in the forms of cumin, turmeric, and curry powder, seems to inhibit the development of certain cancers. Researchers are also studying the effects of allium vegetables such as garlic, onions, scallions, and leeks in fighting cancer.

As with most foods, herbs are best when you buy them fresh and whole. Some commercially ground and prepared products contain extenders such as bark or stems. Whole herbs and spices keep longer than ground ones, which generally keep for six months at the most. Store herbs and spices in airtight containers, away from heat, humidity, and light. Use the broad side of a knife to crush seeds, or grind them in a seed grinder or small coffee mill. This releases the maximum flavor.

Another advantage to buying fresh herbs and spices is that you can blend your own mixes for greater variety. If you add herbs or spices to a cold dish, allow two hours for the flavors to infuse into the food. And when in doubt about how much to use, remember that less is often more — you can always add more to suit your taste. Herbs and spices should enhance, not dominate, foods.

Add a Flair of Flavor

Try these low-fat flavorings, which you can add during preparation or at the table, to give your favorite foods added zest:

- **Herbs** – oregano, basil, cilantro, dill, thyme, parsley, sage, rosemary

- **Spices** – cinnamon, nutmeg, pepper, paprika

- **Fat-free salad dressing**

- **Fruit-sweetened catsup**

- **Tofu mayonnaise**

- **Reduced-sodium soy sauce**

- **Salsa**

- **Lemon or lime juice**

- **Vinegar**

- **Horseradish**

- **Fresh ginger**

- **Sprinkled butter flavor** (not made with real butter)

- **Red pepper flakes**

- **Sprinkle of fat-free soy cheese**

- **Sodium-free salt substitute**

- **Jelly or fruit preserves**, preferably sweetened with fruit juice

Fresh herbs and spices provide the fullest flavor, though dried products are convenient and easy to use. Remember to read the labels for quantity conversions, since dried herbs and spices are usually more concentrated than fresh ones.

Eating Well When Someone Else Does the Cooking

It's easy to eat right when you plan your own menus and fix your own meals. Then you know exactly what goes into each dish, and what combinations of foods help you meet your nutritional guidelines. Eating at someone else's house or at a restaurant can be significantly more challenging. Here are some tips to make it easier:

- Remind friends and family of your special needs. Offer to share recipes or bring prepared dishes that you can eat and others can share.

- Many fine restaurants now feature vegetarian, low-fat, and "heart-healthy" menus. If this is your first visit to the restaurant, call ahead to find out what foods the restaurant serves and how dishes are prepared. Many restaurants will honor special requests if you make them in advance.

- At a friend's house or in a restaurant, ask for sauces, dressings, gravy, and butter or margarine to be served on the side instead of on the food.

- Choose fresh fruits and vegetables whenever possible.

- Select foods that are broiled, steamed, baked, poached, or lightly sautéed.

Everything in Its Place

An organized kitchen makes cooking easy and fun. When it's easy to get a meal started, you're more likely to fix healthy foods. You also save time and energy in preparation. Put the knives, cutting boards, measuring cups, measuring spoons, wooden spoons, and saucepans that you most commonly use in a convenient place. Arrange other cooking supplies to be within easy reach while you're preparing recipes. When it's time to cook, get all the ingredients and supplies you need out and ready to use.

The equipment you use also makes a difference. These two tips can make preparing and cooking food easier and more consistent, so you get the same results each time:

- Use good-quality nonstick pans. Heavy-duty nonstick pans enable you to cook with little or no fat. Sturdy pans cook food faster by letting you sauté over higher heat without burning the food.

- Let modern technology come to your aid in the kitchen. Use a food processor to chop onions, garlic, and fresh herbs and to shred cabbage, carrots, and other vegetables. A mini food processor is ideal for mincing small amounts of garlic, parsley, or other herbs and seasonings. Use a blender to make delicious shakes, smoothies, and other drinks. A blender or food processor is also great for puréeing soups and making quick dessert sauces from fruit.

Before You

Begin

As any good cook will tell you, preparation is the foundation for a great meal. Before you start cleaning, cutting, chopping, and mixing, take a few moments to organize your meal. Here are some questions to help you get started with your planning:

- Are you cooking for just yourself, yourself and your spouse, or your entire family or other large gathering?

- Can you prepare extra portions to freeze for quick meals at times when cooking is inconvenient?

- What tastes or textures are you craving? Can you craft your preferences into a single nutritious meal, or do you need to plan a nutritional balance over several meals?

- Do you have all the ingredients you need to prepare your selected food items?

- How much preparation time will you need? If you're making a recipe for the first time or are not usually the cook, plan to allow yourself extra time.

It's a good idea to take a look at the recipes you're planning to prepare, even if they're old favorites. This helps you evaluate your meal's nutritional content, determine what ingredients you need, and figure out how long before mealtime you need to begin your preparations. Consider planning your meals over several days, so when you go grocery shopping you can buy all that you need in a single trip.

What the Dietary Information Means

Dietary information helps you calculate the amounts of vital nutrients your meals and snacks contain. It also helps you monitor and reduce fat intake. This knowledge enables you to plan nutritious, balanced, and prostate-healthy menus.

The nutritional analysis provided for each recipe in this book was calculated using Micro Cookbook Program put out by software publisher IMSI. Generally, the analysis applies to a single serving, based on the number of servings given for each recipe and the amount of each ingredient. If a range is given for the number of servings and/or the amount of an ingredient, the analysis is based on the average of the figures given.

The nutritional analysis does not include optional ingredients or those for which no specific amount is stated. If you use a substitution for an ingredient, you'll have to calculate the dietary information by removing the original ingredient and replacing it with the substitute. Most of the time this isn't worth the effort, though watch out for substitutions that might be higher in fat or sugar (since sugar converts to fat in your body).

About Substitutions

Fat does add flavor and texture to foods. But cutting the fat from your diet doesn't automatically sentence you to bland meals. Use other substances to replace flavors and textures to turn your old favorites into new taste sensations. Herbs and spices bring out the subtleties of many foods. Tofu is a great substitute for cream cheese and sour cream in dressings and dips. Fruit spreads and bean spreads make delicious toppings for toast and sandwiches. When you bake, replace some of the fat with mashed fruit or blended tofu. And puréed vegetables are wonderful for thickening soups and stews.

Here are a few quick and easy taste treats you can whip up in minutes:

- **Seasoned bean spreads** — Mash cooked beans with chopped onions and celery, herbs or spices, and your favorite condiments (such as lemon juice, salsa, mustard, or catsup) to create delicious sandwich spreads. Use these low-fat, high-flavor substitutes instead of peanut butter and tuna or chicken salad made with mayonnaise.

- **Tofu** — Blend low-fat soft or creamy tofu, instead of cream cheese or sour cream, with herbs and lemon juice for a delightful dip. Blend low-fat tofu, in place of cream or milk, with cooked vegetables to make a rich sauce you can serve over rice or pasta.

- **Egg substitutes** — Replace one egg with 1/4 cup mashed bananas, applesauce, or puréed prunes in cakes and muffins (also add 1/2 teaspoon of baking powder for each egg you leave out of the recipe). Or mix two tablespoons white flour, 1/2 teaspoon olive oil, two tablespoons water, and 1/2 teaspoon of baking powder for each egg you want to replace.

■ **Binders** — In vegetarian cooking, you might find you need something to help hold together the ingredients in a veggie burger mixture or a bean and grain loaf. Try mashed potatoes, tomato paste, flour, matzo meal, or quick oats.

Eating Your Way to
Prostate Health

▼

You can make remarkable changes in your life and your health simply by changing your eating habits. A low-fat, plant-based diet can be both delicious and nutritious, and it can save your life. You can learn new ways to cook your favorite recipes without fat, and with essential soy products and cruciferous vegetables.

The Prostate Diet should reflect your particular preferences. While you must incorporate the general recommendations I've included here, it's important that you plan meals and menus to accommodate your own personal tastes.

Eating should, and can, be more than simply filling your stomach. The food choices you make shape your life and your health. Make your choices count as you enjoy these recipes for your eating pleasure and for your good health!

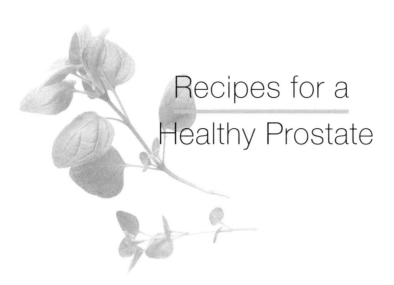

Recipes for a
Healthy Prostate

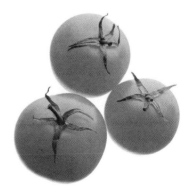

Appetizers and
Snacks

▼

What do you do when you just have to have a snack? Sometimes cravings hit between meals, and other times you might want something light to eat. Or you might want to stem the tide of hunger rising in your dinner guests. Nutritious appetizers and snacks can be a delicious dimension of your prostate cancer nutrition plan. Many of these recipes can also serve as tasty side dishes for light meals such as sandwiches or soups. From the simple to the elegant, these recipes are sure to please.

Tofu Dresses Up Your Dips

Mix tofu with your favorite herbs, spices, and seasonings to create dips and dressings that are as delicious as they are low-fat. Use your creations to add flavor to your favorite sandwiches, too.

Crudités

For this dish, use any blend of vegetables you have on hand.

8 SERVINGS

1 cup carrots

1 cup celery

1 cup jicama

1 cup radishes

1 cup cherry tomatoes

1 cup broccoli, blanched with florets separated

1 cup cauliflower, blanched with florets separated

½ cup snow peas, strings removed

½ cup string beans

Clean the vegetables and cut them into bite-size pieces. Arrange attractively on a serving platter and serve with the low-fat dip of your choice on the side.

Amount Per Serving

Calories 37   Calories from Fat 3   Total Calories From: Fat 7% Protein 17% Carb. 76%

Vitamin A 85%   Vitamin C 65%   Iron 4%

Fruit Kebabs

This is a great snack, a healthy dessert, a breakfast treat along with muffins, or a side dish on your luncheon platter. I like to serve fruit kebabs garnished with lime wedges.

6 SERVINGS

6 12-inch wooden skewers

1 cup cantaloupe, cubed

1 cup pineapple, cubed

1 cup papaya, cubed

1 cup watermelon, cubed

12 strawberries, hulled

2 kiwis, cubed

Thread the fruit on each skewer. Serve chilled.

You can substitute other fruit, depending on what is in season and readily available, such as apples, oranges, peaches, various other melons, etc.

Amount Per Serving

Calories 72   Calories from Fat 5   Total Calories From: Fat 7% Protein 6% Carb. 87%

Vitamin A 22%   Vitamin C 125%   Iron 2%

Savory Edamame

(Whole Green Soybeans in the Pod)

3 SERVINGS

1 pound fresh or frozen edamame (green soybeans in the pod)

sea salt or salt substitute, to taste

1. Simmer the beans in their pods for 5-8 minutes.

2. Drain soybeans, then rinse under cold running water.

3. Sprinkle with salt to taste.

To eat as a snack, open the pods and push out the cooked beans. Provide a bowl to discard the pods.

To serve as a side dish, push out the beans and discard the pods. Season with chopped onions, chives, cumin, curry, rosemary, or thyme. You can also add the cooked beans to soups or salads.

Amount Per Serving

Calories 100   Calories from Fat 30   Total Calories From: Fat 30% Protein 37% Carb. 33%

Vitamin A 6%   Vitamin C 8%   Iron 15%

Tortilla Chips

This is a delicious treat anytime.

4 SERVINGS

1 12-ounce package fat free tortillas

1. Cut tortillas into small triangles. Lay flat on an ungreased cookie sheet. Bake in preheated 350° F oven for 8 minutes or until lightly browned.

2. Serve warm with one of the great bean dips (see page 184) or Home-Cooked Salsa (see page 191).

For a variation, substitute whole-wheat pita pockets for the tortillas. Cut the pita pockets into eighths and place on prepared cookie sheet. Proceed as above. To add extra zip, a light sprinkling of onion powder, garlic powder, chili powder, or other seasoning of choice can be sprinkled on top of chips before baking.

Amount Per Serving

Calories 148	Calories from Fat 23	Total Calories From: Fat 16% Protein 9% Carb. 75%
		Vitamin A 0% Vitamin C 0% Iron 0%

Pita Chips

This is great with any dip!

6 SERVINGS

extra-virgin olive oil cooking spray
1 package pita bread, whole wheat
granulated onion or garlic, to taste

1. Preheat oven to 400° F.

2. Lightly spray a nonstick baking pan with extra-virgin olive oil cooking spray.

3. Cut pita pockets into eighths, and place on prepared pan. Lightly spray the top side of the pita bread and sprinkle with granulated onion or garlic. Bake 9-10 minutes. Place under the broiler about 4 minutes or until lightly browned.

4. Serve immediately with your favorite dip or salsa.

Amount Per Serving

Calories 17   Calories from Fat 1   Total Calories From: Fat 5% Protein 15% Carb. 80%

Vitamin A 0%   Vitamin C 0%   Iron 0%

Baked Potato Chips

The chips take 2 to 2½ hours to bake, so plan ahead. They achieve crispness without added fat, and are delicious!

SERVINGS

½ pound red or white thin-skinned potatoes, unpeeled

½ pound sweet potatoes

extra-virgin olive oil cooking spray

1 teaspoon sea salt or salt substitute

1 teaspoon garlic powder

1. Cut potatoes into very thin slices with a sharp knife. In a 4-quart pan, bring 2 quarts water to a boil. Add potatoes, about a third at a time for about 1½ minutes (until slightly translucent). Lift out with a slotted spoon and drain on paper towels.

2. Place wire racks on 4 large baking sheets. Lightly coat racks with cooking spray.

3. Arrange potato slices on racks in a single layer. Mix the sea salt and garlic powder together. Season the sliced potatoes to taste with garlic salt mixture. Bake in a 200° F oven for approximately 2 to 2½ hours (until chips are crisped).

4. Remove from oven and serve hot or at room temperature.

If you make the chips ahead, let them cool and store in an airtight container at room temperature for up to 1 week.

Amount Per Serving

Calories 81   Calories from Fat 1   Total Calories From: Fat 1% Protein 9% Carb. 90%

Vitamin A 0%   Vitamin C 19%   Iron 5%

Dilly Dill Dip

This is a delicious treat anytime. I recommend you double the recipe and spoon some into baked potatoes at your next meal.

8 SERVINGS

8 ounces low-fat silken soft tofu

¼ cup mellow white miso

2 tablespoons extra-virgin olive oil

1 clove shallot, peeled

1 teaspoon honey

a few sprigs fresh baby dill weed

1. Drain tofu and place in blender with other ingredients, except the dill. Cover and blend until smooth.

2. Garnish with fresh dill sprigs.

3. Serve with raw, crisp vegetables, spread on warm toast, or serve with Baked Potato Chips (see page 47).

Amount Per Serving

Calories 52   Calories from Fat 35   Total Calories From: Fat 67% Protein 8% Carb. 25%

Vitamin A 2%   Vitamin C 0%   Iron 1%

Wowee! Garlic Vegetable Dip

Lots of bite! If we all have garlic at the same time, it's OKAY! I sometimes like to mince all ingredients together by hand rather than in the food processor or blender so it has a chunkier consistency. Either way, it's a winner!

20 SERVINGS

2 cups garlic (approximately 10 heads)

½ teaspoon extra-virgin olive oil

10 jalapeño peppers

1 cup scallions, finely minced

¼ cup lime juice, freshly squeezed

4 tablespoons fish sauce (see glossary)

1. Preheat your oven to 375° F.

2. Cut the top off the garlic heads and drizzle olive oil over top. Put the garlic and jalapeño peppers on a cookie sheet sprayed with olive oil cooking spray. Bake the garlic and jalapeños at 375° F for 35-45 minutes. Remove from oven and let cool at room temperature.

3. Squeeze the garlic cloves from the head and put it into your blender or food processor. Taking a sharp paring knife, gently pull the loosened skin from the jalapeño pepper and discard the skin. Add the jalapeño pepper and all remaining ingredients to the blender or food processor and blend until smooth.

4. Serve on toasted bread, crackers, or as a dip for Crudités (see page 42).

Amount Per Serving

Calories 69   Calories from Fat 4   Total Calories From: Fat 5% Protein 25% Carb. 70%

Vitamin A 8%   Vitamin C 23%   Iron 7%

Vita-Veggie Dip

This dip is best made in the summer when the vegetables are at their finest. I like the squash picked when it is still young and tender.

12 SERVINGS

2 cups onions, chopped

½ teaspoon sea salt
or salt substitute

½ teaspoon of freshly milled
black pepper, or to taste

¼ teaspoon thyme

½ teaspoon basil

2 cloves garlic, minced

1½ cups broccoli, chopped

1 cup yellow summer squash,
chopped

1 green bell pepper, chopped

½ cup pitted black olives,
finely minced

Place all ingredients in a blender or food processor and blend until smooth. Chill for 1 hour before serving. Garnish with a fresh basil leaf or a sprig of thyme.

Amount Per Serving

Calories 28   Calories from Fat 7   Total Calories From: Fat 20% Protein 13% Carb. 67%

Vitamin A 5%   Vitamin C 320%   Iron 3%

Onion Dip

This is a tofu version of the popular dry onion soup mix dip. Serve with Crudités (see page 42) or one of the great low-fat chips in this book (see page 45–47).

6 SERVINGS

**1 10½ ounce package
low-fat silken tofu**

1 package onion soup mix

Mix all ingredients and serve chilled.

Amount Per Serving

Calories 20	Calories from Fat 3	Total Calories From: Fat 17% Protein 15% Carb. 68%
		Vitamin A 0% Vitamin C 0% Iron 1%

Herbed Tofu-Olive Tidbits

Simple to prepare and bursting with flavor, these tasty tidbits hit the spot at any party.

20 SERVINGS

8 ounces firm tofu

2 tablespoons lemon juice

1 teaspoon Dijon mustard

2 tablespoons red wine vinegar

2 tablespoons fresh mint, minced

2 tablespoons fresh chives, minced

2 tablespoons fresh parsley, minced

⅓ cup pitted Kalamata olives, finely chopped

freshly milled black pepper, to taste

sea salt or salt substitute, to taste

2 7-inch whole-wheat pitas
 or 4 7-inch chapatis

1 small red bell pepper, seeded and sliced into thin lengthwise strips

1 small carrot, cut into thin lengthwise strips

1 small cucumber, cut into thin lengthwise strips

1. Mash tofu in a bowl with a fork. Add lemon juice, mustard, and vinegar. Mash well. Mix in mint, chives, parsley and olives. Season to taste with black pepper and salt. Set aside.

2. Cut around outer edge of each pita round to separate into 2 disks. Cut off edges to make each disk into a square.

3. Warm pitas by placing in a hot skillet for 10-15 seconds on each side.
Spread ¼ of tofu mixture on each square. About 1 inch from one edge, place rows of red pepper, carrot, and cucumber strips. Gently press into tofu. Firmly roll up each square to form a cylinder.

4. With a sharp knife, slice each cylinder crosswise into 4 or 5 pieces. Place a toothpick in each to hold it firmly together. Stand each cylinder on the cut edge to serve.

Amount Per Serving

Calories 22   Calories from Fat 12   Total Calories From: Fat 56% Protein 22% Carb. 22%

Vitamin A 13%   Vitamin C 12%   Iron 5%

Tomato-Caper Bruschetta

This is a nice treat when you have friends over, you're sitting around chatting, and want a quick, easy snack.

8 SERVINGS

1 cup sun-dried tomatoes,
 firmly packed (not in oil)

6 Whole Wheat Baguettes
(see page 214)

3 green onions including tops

2 cloves garlic, minced

1 tablespoon capers, drained

1 tablespoon fresh oregano

1½ tablespoons fresh lemon juice

1 tablespoon balsamic vinegar

sea salt or salt substitute, to taste

1. Combine tomatoes with 1 cup boiling water and set aside until soft and pliable, about 15 minutes. Drain tomatoes.

2. While tomatoes are set aside, cut baguettes diagonally into 24 slices. Arrange on a baking sheet. Broil 4 to 6 inches from heat until toasted on each side, about 2 minutes total.

3. In a food processor or blender, finely mince tomatoes, onions, garlic, capers, and oregano with lemon juice and balsamic vinegar. Add salt to taste.

4. Spoon tomato mixture into a small bowl and accompany with baguette slices. Spread tomato mixture on slices to eat.

Amount Per Serving

Calories 37   Calories from Fat 4   Total Calories From: Fat 11% Protein 13% Carb. 76%

Vitamin A 0%   Vitamin C 7%   Iron 3%

Napa Cabbage Rolls

A great appetizer with the traditional flavors of China.

6 SERVINGS

olive oil cooking spray

1 bunch Napa cabbage

2 green bell peppers, cut into julienne strips

2 tablespoons tamari soy sauce

2 tablespoons malt vinegar

2 ½ tablespoons rice syrup

½ teaspoon sea salt or salt substitute

¼ teaspoon crushed dried chili peppers

1. Separate Napa cabbage into single leaves. Boil cabbage leaves in lightly salted water until just barely tender, usually about 10 minutes, then drain carefully and rinse with running cold water.

2. Cut each leaf crosswise into 2 parts, and when cool roll tightly. Then cut each roll into 1-inch strips. Arrange the cabbage rolls in a shallow serving dish.

3. Spray a nonstick skillet with olive oil cooking spray and sauté the green peppers over medium-high heat for 3 minutes. Add remaining ingredients, mix well, and cook for a minute or two longer, then pour the mixture over the cabbage rolls.

4. Let stand at room temperature for 30 minutes or so before serving.

Amount Per Serving

Calories 31   Calories from Fat 3   Total Calories From: Fat 8% Protein 29% Carb. 63%

Vitamin A 72%   Vitamin C 122%   Iron 6%

Toi's Mock Thai Chicken Salad

A friend from Thailand visited us and made the traditional version of this dish using chicken breast. It was an instant hit. This is my variation on that traditional recipe. It's easy to make and is a great snack anytime. Don't be surprised if it becomes a family favorite!

6 SERVINGS

⅞ cup water

1 cup textured vegetable protein (see glossary)

2 tablespoons brown rice, uncooked

1 teaspoon freshly ground chili powder, or to taste

4 tablespoons fresh lime juice

2 tablespoons fish sauce, or to taste (see glossary)

1 teaspoon fresh galangal, finely minced (see glossary)

pinch of sugar

1 head Napa cabbage

1. Boil the water in a small saucepan. Put the textured vegetable protein in a bowl. Pour the boiling water over the textured vegetable protein, cover, and let it rest for 10 minutes.

2. Heat a heavy-bottomed skillet over high heat. Place rice in the skillet, lower heat to medium, and cook the rice, stirring constantly, until the rice is slightly browned, approximately 2 minutes.
Remove rice from heat and coarsely grind. I do this in a coffee grinder, which I use just for spices.

3. Mix the rice and remaining ingredients in a small bowl.

4. Add spice mixture to the textured vegetable protein. Microwave for an additional 4 minutes.

5. To serve, place mixture on fresh cabbage leaves and eat as finger food.

For variety, substitute tempeh for the textured vegetable protein. Cut it into small pieces, brown in nonstick skillet, and proceed from step #2 above.

Amount Per Serving

Calories 72   Calories from Fat 0   Total Calories From: Fat 0% Protein 67% Carb. 33%

Vitamin A 1%   Vitamin C 5%   Iron 78%

Stuffed Grape Leaves

My husband loves this dish as a mid-day snack.
It's easy to prepare and easy to grab before you rush out the door.

6 SERVINGS

extra-virgin olive oil cooking spray

1 cup red onions, finely chopped

¼ cup raisins

¼ cup dried apricots, finely chopped

2 tablespoons fresh mint leaves, chopped

¼ teaspoon ground cinnamon

¼ teaspoon ground allspice

½ cup brown rice, cooked

sea salt or salt substitute, to taste

freshly milled black pepper, to taste

14 grape leaves, rinsed of brine and dried

¼ cup fresh lemon juice

mint leaves for garnish

lemon slices for garnish

1. Heat a large nonstick skillet and spray it with olive oil cooking spray. Add onion and cook, stirring often until soft, about 5 minutes. Add water as needed to prevent burning. Remove from heat and add raisins, apricots, mint, cinnamon and allspice. Stir in rice and season with salt and pepper to taste.

2. To fill grape leaves: Place one leaf flat on work surface with veins facing upward. Place 2 teaspoons filling in middle of leaf close to stalk end. Fold bottom of leaf over and each side in to enclose filling. Roll up firmly toward point. Place roll in the palm of hand and give a slight squeeze to form a firm shape. Repeat procedure with remaining leaves and filling.

3. Arrange stuffed leaves, seam sides down, in a medium skillet. Add oil, lemon juice, and enough water to cover leaves. Cover pan and cook over low heat for 1½ to 2 hours or until tender. Add extra water to skillet as necessary.

4. Allow leaves to cool, covered, in skillet. Transfer to a serving dish. Serve garnished with lemon and mint, if desired.

Amount Per Serving

Calories 168   Calories from Fat 9   Total Calories From: Fat 5% Protein 8% Carb. 87%

Vitamin A 13%   Vitamin C 14%   Iron 6%

Lentil-Rice Balls

8 SERVINGS

½ cup brown rice, cooked

½ cup lentils, cooked

1 small sweet potato, peeled, cooked, and minced

6 spinach leaves, rinsed, blanched, and finely shredded

½ cup fresh mushrooms, chopped

1 teaspoon tamari soy sauce

sea salt or salt substitute, to taste

freshly milled black pepper, to taste

¾ cup dried breadcrumbs

1 tablespoon cilantro, finely chopped

extra-virgin olive oil cooking spray

1. Preheat oven to 375° F.

2. Combine rice, lentils, sweet potato, spinach, and mushrooms in a large bowl. Add tamari, salt, and pepper. Add breadcrumbs and cilantro and mix well. Refrigerate for 15 to 30 minutes.

3. Form mixture into balls either by hand or using a melon scoop.

4. Spray a cookie sheet with extra-virgin olive oil and place balls on cookie sheet. Bake for 45 minutes or until heated through and the balls turn a medium brown. Remove from oven and serve with your favorite nonfat sauce.

By forming the lentil-rice mixture into patties instead of balls, you can eat these on buns as a hearty sandwich. Double the batch and freeze half for a quick appetizer when unexpected guests arrive.

Amount Per Serving

Calories 115	Calories from Fat 6	Total Calories From: Fat 5%	Protein 20%	Carb. 75%
		Vitamin A 122%	Vitamin C 27%	Iron 14%

Lemon Tofu

Ward likes these as a snack any time of the day.
I like to serve fresh fruit alongside the tofu.

4 SERVINGS

1 pound firm tofu

1 teaspoon organic lemon zest

3 tablespoons fresh lemon juice

3 tablespoons soy sauce

1½ tablespoons onions, finely chopped

2 cloves garlic, pressed or minced

1 tablespoon ginger root, peeled and grated

1. Cut the tofu into 8 slices and arrange in one layer in a glass pan.

2. Mix the remaining ingredients together and pour the mixture over the tofu. Marinate from 3 to 12 hours.

3. Preheat the broiler and broil 3 minutes on each side until browned.

4. Serve piping hot from the broiler or at room temperature.

Amount Per Serving

Calories 110   Calories from Fat 49   Total Calories From: Fat 44% Protein 37% Carb. 19%

Vitamin A 2%   Vitamin C 11%   Iron 36%

Sweet 'n Spicy Apple Butter

Use this delicious spread on bread, muffins, and pancakes.

12 SERVINGS

12 ounces unsweetened applesauce

½ cup concentrated apple juice

1 tablespoon cornstarch

¼ teaspoon ground ginger

pinch of ground cloves

¼ teaspoon nutmeg, freshly ground

4 teaspoons cinnamon

2 teaspoons vanilla extract

1. In a nonstick saucepan cook first 7 ingredients until mixture thickens. Continue to simmer for 5 minutes.

2. Remove from heat, and stir in vanilla. Store in refrigerator until ready to use.

Amount Per Serving

Calories 36	Calories from Fat 1	Total Calories From: Fat 3% Protein 1% Carb. 96%
		Vitamin A 0% Vitamin C 9% Iron 3%

Fruity Marinade

Tofu and tempeh can be treated as meat when marinated. You can grill, broil, or stir-fry the tofu fillets in the same way that many cuts of meat are prepared. You can thread them on skewers with vegetables or pineapple, sauté chunks and use them in many of your favorite salads, or in sandwiches.

2 CUPS

1½ cups apple juice,
or other fruit juice, such as orange

⅓ cup tamari soy sauce

2 tablespoons lemon juice
or apple cider vinegar

2 tablespoons ginger root,
peeled and freshly grated

2 cloves garlic, pressed or minced

1 teaspoon toasted sesame oil

a few dashes of cayenne pepper

Put all ingredients in blender and blend until smooth. Use as a marinade for either tofu or tempeh.

Amount Per Serving

Calories 180   Calories from Fat 6   Total Calories From: Fat 4% Protein 20% Carb. 76%

Vitamin A 2%   Vitamin C 43%   Iron 13%

Beans, Grains, and Vegetable Basics

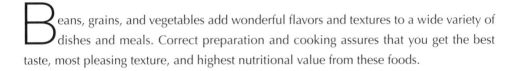

Beans, grains, and vegetables add wonderful flavors and textures to a wide variety of dishes and meals. Correct preparation and cooking assures that you get the best taste, most pleasing texture, and highest nutritional value from these foods.

Beans (Legumes)

Buy beans at a store that has a rapid turnover of dried beans, and use them within a few months. If your beans are older than six months, they will take much longer to cook until tender. A tender bean is one that you can mash on the roof of your mouth with your tongue. Buying canned, cooked beans is fine when you're in a hurry. But be sure to read labels carefully. Choose organic products and products that don't contain unwanted ingredients such as preservatives, MSG, or high amounts of sodium. Cooking your own beans is much less expensive than buying canned beans and the taste is fresher. And flavorings such as garlic, chili peppers, and onions are more deeply absorbed if you add them during cooking. Remember that you can cook a big batch of beans and freeze part of it for another day and another recipe.

Cleaning Beans

Though fragments of stems, sticks, and small stones remind you that your beans are natural, they can be unpleasant surprises when they slip through to your cooked dishes. Sort and clean your beans to prepare them for cooking. The most efficient way to do this is to measure the beans and spread them out on a cookie sheet or a large flat baking pan. Starting at the top, quickly brush the beans towards the top of the sheet, picking out sticks, stones, and dried-out or dead-looking beans as you go. Then pour the good beans into a colander (strainer) and rinse them thoroughly to remove any dirt.

Soaking Beans

After you clean and rinse your beans, soak them overnight to soften them. This speeds cooking time and makes the beans easier to digest. The water draws the indigestible carbohydrates out, leaving the nutrients. When you're ready to cook the beans, drain and discard the soaking water and rinse them again with fresh water.

If you don't have a lot of time for soaking, follow this recipe for a quick-soak method: Rinse and sort the beans. Place 1 cup of beans in cooking pot with 3½ to 4 cups of water. Bring water to a rolling boil and immediately remove beans from the heat, allowing them to stand, covered, for 1 hour. Cook per recipe instructions.

Cooking Beans

Most beans take time to cook—how much time depends on the kind of beans. Small beans such as lentils are done in about half an hour, while larger beans such as soybeans and garbanzos (chickpeas) take up to four hours. Pressure-cooking gives beans a creamy texture and deep flavor, and also reduces cooking time. An electric slow cooker takes longer, but lets you cook beans while you work or sleep. If you want beans for salads, cook by simmering rather than pressure-cooking, and salt them when they reach the stage you want. Salting them keeps the outer layer from becoming soft and mushy.

Always salt beans at the end of cooking time. You can use a salt substitute if you're concerned about too much sodium in your diet. Salting toughens the outer layer and if you salt the beans early you will have tough beans. Beans need a lot of salt to bring up the flavor. For one cup of dry beans, add at least one teaspoon of salt or salt substitute after they are cooked.

Grains

Buy whole grains at the grocery store or health food market. Shorten the cooking time of grains by soaking them first to soften them, or try toasting them in a slow oven to bring out their natural nutty flavor. Combine longer-cooking grains, such as barley and wild rice, with shorter-cooking grains, such as millet and quinoa, to create exciting and varied tastes and textures. And cook extra quantities that you can use for quick leftover meals and second-day salads.

Vegetables

Buy the freshest vegetables you can find, or grow your own. Natural food stores and consumer cooperatives feature vegetables and fruits grown without pesticides. Some supermarkets also have good produce sections. Scrub or peel vegetables before eating or cooking to remove dirt and bacteria.

Most cooked vegetables taste and look best when they are hot and tender, but not limp and colorless. Steaming is a fast way to cook vegetables and still preserve their valuable nutrients. Though frozen vegetables are convenient, their nutritional value is less than half that of fresh vegetables—and canned vegetables have virtually no nutritional value whatsoever.

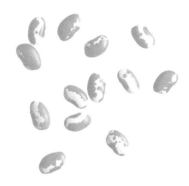

Cooking Times and Proportions for Beans

Type of Bean (1 cup dry)	Amount of Water or Broth	Stove Top (unsoaked)	Stove Top (soaked)	Pressure Cooker (unsoaked)	Pressure Cooker (soaked)	Crockpot on high (soaked)	Yield
Adzuki	3 cups	2 hours	45-60 min	15-20 min	10-15 min	8-12 hours	2 cups
Black Bean	3-4 cups	2 hours	1½ hours	20-25 min	15-20 min	8-10 hours	2 cups
Black-Eyed Pea	3 cups	45-60 min	30-45 min	10-15 min	NR	6-8 hours	2 cups
Garbanzo Beans (Chickpeas)	4 cups	2½-3 hours	1½-2 hours	30-40 min	20-25 min	12-16 hours	2 cups
Great Northern or Navy Beans	3-4 cups	1½-2 hours	1-1½ hours	25-30 min	15-20 min	8-12 hours	2 cups
Kidney	3 cups	2-2½ hours	1-1½ hours	20-25 min	15-20 min	16 hours	2 cups
Lentil (whole Brown/Green)	3 cups	45 min	15-20 min	NR	NR	4-5 hours	2½ cups
Lentils (Red)	3 cups	15-30 min	NR	NR	NR	NR	2½ cups
Lima	2 cups	1½-2 hours	1 hour	15-20 min	10-15 min	8-12 hours	1½ cups
Mung	3 cups	1½ hours	1 hour	15-20 min	10-15 min	8-10 hours	2 cups
Pinto	3 cups	1½-2 hours	1-1½ hours	20-25 min	10-15 min	8-12 hours	2 cups
Soy	4 cups	3-4 hours	2-3 hours	NR	NR	24-48 hours	2 cups
Split Peas	3-4 cups	50-60 min	30 min	NR	NR	8-10 hours	2½ cups

NR = Not Recommended.   Soaked = 8-12 hours presoaked in refrigerator, or boil 5 minutes and soak 2 hours. Unsoaked beans may require double the amount of liquid listed and far longer cooking times. **Pressure cooker:** Set on high (15 lbs. Pressure). Timing begins when full pressure is reached. **Crockpot:** Presoak as above. Exact lengths of cooking times for beans vary greatly by every method, depending on age and quality of beans, as well as amount of liquid used and other variables.

Legume Flavoring Chart

	Adzuki	Black Bean	Black Eyed Pea	Chick Pea	Kidney	Lentil	Lima	Navy	Pinto	Soy	YellowPea
Allspice	*	*		*		*	*	*		*	*
Basil	*	*	*	*		*	*	*		*	*
Bay Leaf	*	*	*	*	*	*	*	*	*	*	*
Caraway			*	*	*			*	*		
Celery Seed		*				*					
Chives	*	*		*		*	*	*	*	*	*
Cilantro	*	*	*	*	*	*	*	*	*	*	*
Cinnamon			*		*				*		
Currants	*			*		*		*		*	*
Curry	*					*				*	
Garlic	*	*	*	*	*	*	*	*		*	*
Ginger	*	*	*	*	*	*	*	*	*	*	*
Lemon		*	*		*				*		
Mace			*		*		*		*		
Mint	*	*		*		*	*	*	*	*	*
Miso	*	*		*		*	*	*		*	*
Mustard	*	*	*	*	*	*	*	*		*	*
Onion	*	*		*		*	*	*		*	
Oregano	*	*	*	*	*	*	*	*		*	*
Paprika			*		*				*		
Parsley	*	*	*	*	*	*	*	*		*	*
Rosemary	*	*	*	*	*	*		*	*	*	
Saffron			*	*	*				*		
Sage	*	*		*		*	*	*		*	*
Savory			*	*	*			*			
Tamari	*	*		*		*	*	*		*	*
Thyme	*	*	*	*		*	*	*		*	*

Cooking Times and Proportions for Grains

Type of Grain	Amount of Grain	Amount of Liquid	Cooking Time (unsoaked, stovetop)	Yield
Amaranth	1 cup	2 cups	30 min	2 cups
Barley, hulled or hull-less	1 cup	2½–3 cups	1–1½ hours	2 cups
Bulgur (cooked, dried, cracked wheat) for dinner grain	1 cup	2 cups	10 min	3 cups
Bulgur (cooked, dried, cracked wheat) for salads	1 cup	2 cups boiling	30 min, soaking only	3 cups
Couscous, whole durum wheat	1 cup	2 cups boiling	5 min, soaking only	2 cups
Millet, for dinner grain	1 cup	2 cups	20–30 min	3 cups
Millet, for porridge or pudding	1 cup	4 cups (part fruit juice)	45–60 min	3 cups
Quinoa	1 cup	2 cups	10 min	4 cups
Rice, Basmati or Texmati, brown	1 cup	2 cups	45 min	3 cups
Rice, brown long	1 cup	1½–2 cups	45–60 min	3 cups
Rice, brown short	1 cup	2–2½	45–60 min	3 cups
Rice, brown sweet glutinous (sticky)	1 cup	2 cups	45–60 min	3 cups
Rice mix (Country Wild™)	1 cup	2 cups	45–60 min	3 cups
Rice, wild	1 cup	3 cups	40–50 min	3 cups
Rolled grains, mixed or single	1 cup	2½–3 cups	15–30 min	2 cups
Rolled oats, regular or thick	1 cup	2–2½ cups	5–15 min	2 cups
Teff	1 cup	2½ cups	20 min	2 cups
Whole grains (kamut, oats, rye, spelt, triticale, wheat)	1 cup	2–3 cups	1–2 hr	2–4 cups

Note: Large grains can be pressure-cooked. Use about ½ cup less liquid and reduce the cooking time by half.

Grain Flavoring Chart

	Barley	Bulgur	Couscous	Millet	Quinoa	BrownRice	BasmatiRice	Rye
Allspice	*							
Anise					*			
Bay Leaf		*	*	*		*	*	*
Cardamon	*							
Chives							*	*
Cilantro		*						*
Cinnamon	*					*		
Clove	*		*					
Coriander						*		
Currants	*						*	
Curry						*	*	
Fennel					*			
Garlic	*	*	*		*	*	*	
Ginger	*			*				
Mace	*				*			
Mint	*							
Nutmeg	*							
Onion			*	*	*	*	*	
Parsley		*	*	*	*	*	*	*
Saffron						*	*	
Sage						*	*	
Tarragon		*	*		*			
Thyme					*	*		
Turmeric			*					
Sake					*	*		
Rice Vinegar		*	*	*	*	*	*	*
Tamari		*	*	*	*	*	*	*

Small Bean Basics

(no soaking required)

The small bean family includes adzuki beans, mung beans, black-eyed peas, green or yellow split peas, and red, green, or brown lentils. I suggest that beans be cooked with kelp, as it tenderizes beans. Kelp also adds minerals to the beans. Small beans do not require presoaking.

6 SERVINGS

2 cups small dried beans

4 – 5 cups water

2 ½-inch piece of kombu

sea salt or salt substitute, to taste

1. Rinse and drain the beans. Place beans, water, and kombu in a 4 quart pot. Bring to a boil. Reduce heat, cover, and simmer.

2. Most of the small beans take 45-55 minutes to cook. Adzuki beans, however, take an hour, and red lentils only take about 20 minutes.

3. Add the salt at the end of cooking time.

Amount Per Serving

Calories 124   Calories from Fat 1   Total Calories From: Fat 1% Protein 29% Carb. 70%

Vitamin A 0%   Vitamin C 3%   Iron 19%

Big Bean Basics

(soaking required)

Cannelloni, garbanzo (chickpeas), black, great northern, kidney, lima, and pinto are some of the more popular varieties of big beans. Kombu (a sea vegetable), also known as kelp, is added to tenderize the beans. Kombu also adds minerals to the cooking beans.

6 SERVINGS

2 cups beans, dried

6 cups water

**2½ inch piece of kombu,
soaked 10 minutes in cold water**

1 teaspoon sea salt or salt substitute

1. Sort and clean the beans. Soak beans 8-12 hours or overnight.

2. Drain off and discard soaking water. Put soaked beans, fresh water, and kombu in a pot. Bring to a boil. Lower heat and simmer, covered, until beans are quite tender, about 60 minutes. A well-cooked bean can be mashed easily on the roof of the mouth with the tongue. Add water during cooking if needed.

3. Salt beans at the end of the cooking time after they have softened.

Amount Per Serving

Calories 124	Calories from Fat 1	Total Calories From: Fat 1% Protein 29% Carb. 70%
		Vitamin A 0% Vitamin C 3% Iron 19%

Slow-Cooked Beans

Soak beans overnight or by quick-soak method (see page 62). Drain off and discard soaking water, then follow directions that apply to your slow cooker. This is typically 8 hours on at the highest temperature.

Pressure-Cooked Beans

Two cups of dried beans make about 6 cups of cooked beans.

8 SERVINGS

2 cups dried beans, soaked

4 cups water

**3-inch piece of kombu,
soaked 5 minutes in cold water**

1 teaspoon sea salt or salt substitute

Drain off and discard soaking water. Rinse beans. Put beans, fresh water, and kombu in pressure cooker. Attach lid. Bring up to pressure on medium heat. You should hear a soft hissing sound. Lower heat and let beans cook 40-45 minutes. Remove from heat and allow pressure to come down naturally or run cold water over the top of the cooker. Add salt after cooking.

Brown Rice Basics

Rice with just the hull removed is brown rice. Rice with the hull, bran, and germ removed is white rice. Brown rice comes in a variety of types: short grain, long grain, and Basmati are three common varieties. All can be prepared in the same manner.

6 SERVINGS

1 cup brown rice, uncooked
pinch of sea salt or salt substitute
1¾ – 2 cups water

Rinse and drain rice. Place rice in a pot with salt and water. Bring to a boil. Turn heat to low. Cover the pot and let the rice simmer for about 45 minutes or until all the water is absorbed. Don't stir the rice while it is cooking. Not only is it unnecessary, but stirring the grain as it cooks or comes to boil will cause the starches to separate, preventing steam from rising up and cooking the grain evenly. Stirring grain as it cooks leads to sticky grain and burned pots. Do not stir, and do not lift the lid or steam will escape. The boiling water will do all the stirring necessary leaving you free to do other things while your grain cooks.

Amount Per Serving

Calories 113   Calories from Fat 8   Total Calories From: Fat 7% Protein 9% Carb. 84%

Vitamin A 0%   Vitamin C 0%   Iron 3%

Bulgur Basics

Bulgur is par-boiled, dried, and cracked whole wheat. It can be used as a base grain for a variety of bean and vegetable dishes, including tabouli, a traditional Middle-Eastern dish.

6 SERVINGS

1 cup water

pinch of sea salt or salt substitute

1 cup bulgur

Bring water and salt to a boil in a small pan. Add bulgur. Remove from heat and cover pan. Fluff the grain with a fork before serving. Add a few drops of olive oil to the cooked bulgur to keep it loose.

Amount Per Serving

Calories 85	Calories from Fat 3	Total Calories From: Fat 3% Protein 13% Carb. 84%
Vitamin A 0%	Vitamin C 0%	Iron 3%

Basic Rolled Oats

Oat groats that have been heated until soft and pressed flat are called rolled oats, whereas oat groats that have been thinly sliced are called steel-cut oats. You use the same technique for cooking both.

6 SERVINGS

1 cup rolled oats

pinch of sea salt or salt substitute

3 cups water

Place oats in a pot with salt and water. Bring to a boil, reduce heat, cover, and let simmer on low heat for 20-25 minutes. If you wish to spice up the oats by adding raisins and/or cinnamon, do this during the last 10 minutes of cooking.

Amount Per Serving

Calories 52   Calories from Fat 8   Total Calories From: Fat 15% Protein 16% Carb. 69%

Vitamin A 0%   Vitamin C 0%   Iron 3%

Basic Quinoa

Quinoa is a delicious grain that comes from the Andes Mountains in South America. When quinoa is cooked, it opens up to make tiny spirals. It contains all 8 amino acids and therefore has better protein value than most grains.

6 SERVINGS

1 cup quinoa

pinch of sea salt or salt substitute

1¾ cups water

Rinse quinoa well with warm water and drain. Place rinsed quinoa, salt, and water in a pot. Bring to a boil, reduce heat to low, cover, and let simmer 15-20 minutes, until all the water is absorbed. Fluff with a fork before serving.

Amount Per Serving

Calories 108   Calories from Fat 15   Total Calories From: Fat 14% Protein 14% Carb. 72%

Vitamin A 0%   Vitamin C 0%   Iron 15%

Cooking Whole-Grain Noodles and Pasta

4 SERVINGS

**8 ounces of any whole-grain pasta
(eggless or made with the whites only)**

**½ – 1 teaspoon sea salt
or salt substitute**

¼ teaspoon of extra-virgin olive oil

Choose a pot large enough to give the noodles plenty of room to dance; an 8-quart pot works well. Fill pot with water and bring to a boil. Add salt and oil. Drop the noodles in slowly. To prevent sticking, stir the noodles gently with a wooden spoon for the first few minutes. Follow package directions for cooking time. Test noodles for doneness by eating one. You are aiming for a tender yet firm noodle that is chewy. Put cooked noodles in a colander and rinse well. Let them drain well, as excess moisture can lead to mushiness.

Soups, Sandwiches,
and Salads

▼

When you're hungry, you want something good and nutritious…now. Soups, sandwiches, and salads offer quick fixings for fast meals. Combine a soup or sandwich and a salad for a delicious and satisfying lunch. Serve soup as an appetizer, or salad with a main dish for dinner. Salads, with their abundance of fresh, raw vegetables, are especially valuable as part of The Prostate Diet. Only your imagination limits the possibilities to mix and match selections from these recipes for meals as light or as hearty as your appetite.

Leftovers Make Tasty Light Meals

It's easy and healthy to whip up a quick lunch with leftovers. Combine your favorites with a salad and fresh bread, and you have a nutritious, tasty meal with almost no effort.

Basic Vegetable Stock

Homemade soup stock gives any soup a special, rich flavor. You can vary this recipe according to the vegetables available in your garden or refrigerator. Save the ends and bits whenever you cut vegetables (tops of celery, parsley, stems, etc.) to include in this recipe.

3 tablespoons water for sautéing

2 onions, or 1 onion and 1 leek

4 cloves garlic, minced

1 inch round of ginger root, peeled, smashed and chopped

2 cups celery

1 cup carrots

1 cup turnips or potatoes

2 shiitake mushrooms

6 sprigs fresh parsley

2 sprigs fresh thyme, or 1 teaspoon dried

1 teaspoon freshly ground black pepper

2 bay leaves

8 cups cold water

1. Coarsely chop all vegetables into 1-inch chunks (if you scrub the vegetables, there is no need to peel them). Pour 3 tablespoons water into large stockpot over medium heat. Add the onion and sauté for 5 minutes, stirring often. Add the garlic and continue sautéing for an additional 3 minutes. Letting the onions get brown on the bottom and debraising the stockpot with a little water adds flavor.

2. Add the rest of the ingredients and cook for an additional 4 minutes. Cover with water, bring to a boil, reduce heat, and simmer for 45 minutes.

3. Strain the stock and throw away the vegetables. Store the stock in your refrigerator up to one week or freeze for later use.

I often make really simple stocks at a moment's notice by combining only two or three vegetables such as:

- Parsnips and leeks
- Broccoli and onion
- Butternut squash, onion, and celery

For Asian soup stock, I often put vegetables from the cruciferous family, along with onions and garlic, into a large roasting pan with enough water to cover and bake at 300° F for approximately 3 hours.

(If you're in a hurry and don't have any of this delicious homemade stock on hand, try Vogue Instant Vege Base, which you can find in most health food stores.)

Amount Per Serving

Calories 95	Calories from Fat 5	Total Calories From: Fat 5%	Protein 12%	Carb. 83%
		Vitamin A 160%	Vitamin C 38%	Iron 12%

Garlic Stock

This is a stock, like vegetable stock, used for cooking soups, grains, and beans.

1½ pounds garlic heads,
cut in half crosswise

2 onions

8 cloves

4 carrots, chopped in thirds

2 bay leaves

2 bunches parsley

6 quarts water

1. Place the garlic in an 8-quart soup pot. Stud each onion with 4 cloves by pushing the stem of the cloves into the onion and add to the pot. Add the carrots, bay leaves, parsley bunches, and water. Bring to a boil. Reduce heat to a simmer and cook uncovered for 2½ hours.

2. Strain the stock. Cool and store in the refrigerator for up to 3 days or in the freezer for up to 4 months.

Amount Per Serving

Calories 61   Calories from Fat 3   Total Calories From: Fat 4% Protein 14% Carb. 82%

Vitamin A 1638%   Vitamin C 460%   Iron 102%

Kombu Stock

This stock is great to use when making miso soups. It adds minerals and enhances the flavor of the soup.

1 6-inch kombu strip (see glossary)

8 dried shiitake mushrooms, cleaned and rinsed

2 quarts water

1 bunch scallions, including tops, chopped

1 carrot, thinly sliced

1. Clean the kombu and shiitake mushrooms. Soak them in water until they become tender, approximately 15 minutes.
Drain.

2. Put the shiitake mushrooms and kombu in a large stockpot along with the water and the rest of the ingredients. Bring to a boil, then lower the heat and simmer, covered, for 20 minutes.

3. Strain the stock. You may wish to save the cooked mushrooms to use at a later date in a soup.

This stock will keep for a week in the refrigerator. You can also freeze it in an ice cube tray and transfer each cube to a resealable bag. Keep it frozen up to 3 months to add to soups as needed.

Amount Per Serving

Calories 218   Calories from Fat 4   Total Calories From: Fat 7% Protein 20% Carb. 73%

Vitamin A 406%   Vitamin C 13%   Iron 21%

Stir-Fry Stock

I substitute stir-fry stock for oil in stir-fry recipes. If you freeze the stock in ice cube trays, remove the cubes to a resealable bag. They're easy to use in as little or as large amounts as needed.

8 SERVINGS

1 small onion, finely sliced

4 cloves garlic, minced

2 large carrots, thinly sliced

1 bunch scallions, including tops

6 shiitake mushrooms, cleaned

½ cup chopped cilantro

1 6-inch piece kombu stick
(see glossary)

1 tablespoon tamari soy sauce

1 tablespoon of mirin
(see glossary)

sea salt or salt substitute,
to taste

2 quarter-size slices of ginger root

8 cups cold water

1. Sauté the onion in large stockpot with a small amount of water or nonstick cooking spray for 5 minutes. Add the garlic and sauté for an additional minute. Add all remaining ingredients.

2. Bring to a boil, then lower heat and simmer for 40 minutes.

3. Strain the stock and store it in the refrigerator for up to one week, or it may be frozen for longer use. I like to freeze this stock in my ice cube trays and transfer it to resealable bags so I can use small amounts at a time.

Amount Per Serving

Calories 30   Calories from Fat 1   Total Calories From: Fat 7% Protein 12% Carb. 81%

Vitamin A 127%   Vitamin C 6%   Iron 2%

Cantaloupe Soup

Make sure the melon you use for this recipe is ripe. Vine-ripened is best, but if not available, look for a uniform cream rind color, rather than greenish netting, for ripeness. The stem end should be smooth, slightly depressed, and yield slightly to pressure. Good aroma indicates good flavor. The cantaloupe should feel heavy for its size.

4 SERVINGS

4 cups cantaloupe, cubed

¾ cup orange juice

½ cup low-fat silken tofu

4 mint leaves, for garnish

1. Blend 2 cups cantaloupe, half of the orange juice, and ¼ cup tofu in blender or food processor until smooth. Transfer to large bowl. Repeat with remaining cantaloupe, juice, and tofu.

2. Cover and chill up to 24 hours. Serve garnished with mint leaves.

Amount Per Serving

Calories 101   Calories from Fat 6   Total Calories From: Fat 5% Protein 14% Carb. 81%

Vitamin A 104%   Vitamin C 140%   Iron 2%

Miso Soup with Wakame

This is the most basic style of Japanese miso soups. While any type of miso works, my favorite is a combination of full-flavored dark miso and a mellow light miso. You can find the combo packs in Asian markets.

4 SERVINGS

4 cups water or 2 cups Kombu Stock (see page 81) with 2 cups water

1 ounce wakame leaf (see glossary)

1–3 tablespoons miso, to taste (see glossary)

1 10-ounce package tofu, diced (optional)

2 scallions, thinly sliced, for garnish

1. Break wakame leaves into small pieces, then bring the water or kombu stock to a boil. Add the wakame and simmer for 4 minutes. Add tofu, if using, and simmer for 2 minutes longer.

2. Dilute the miso with ½ cup of the stock. Stir the diluted miso into the pot a little at a time and taste. Add as much as needed to suit your taste. Simmer for 1 minute, making sure the soup does not boil.

3. Divide the sliced scallions into four equal servings and place them into the serving bowls. Pour the miso soup into the bowls. Serve immediately.

Be creative with this soup. Add tofu, or instead of wakame, add daikon (see glossary) or small pieces of thinly sliced potato, onions, and carrots. The combinations are endless.

Amount Per Serving

Calories 28   Calories from Fat 7   Total Calories From: Fat 25% Protein 23% Carb. 52%

Vitamin A 0%   Vitamin C 0%   Iron 2%

Cabbage-Miso Soup

I often substitute garlic stock for the vegetable stock. Experiment to see what suits your taste buds. We enjoy variety and are constantly experimenting with new ways of presenting old favorites.

4 SERVINGS

extra-virgin olive oil cooking spray

1 onion, finely chopped

4 cloves garlic, finely minced

2 cups cabbage, finely shredded

1 cup shiitake mushrooms, thinly sliced

5 cups Basic Vegetable Stock (see page 78)

3 tablespoons tamari soy sauce

3 tablespoons rice vinegar

1 tablespoon molasses

¼ cup cilantro, chopped

4 tablespoons miso (see glossary)

½ teaspoon Red Chili Paste (see page 196)

1. Spray a large nonstick saucepan with olive oil cooking spray and place over medium heat. Add onion and garlic and sauté for 5 minutes or until soft. Add water if needed to prevent burning.

2. Stir in cabbage and cook another 5 minutes. Stir in mushrooms, stock, soy sauce, vinegar, and molasses. Cover and simmer for about 25 minutes or until vegetables are tender.

3. Stir in cilantro, miso, and Red Chili Paste. Be sure not to boil the miso as this deactivates it and negates some of its beneficial effects. Serve immediately.

Amount Per Serving

Calories 145   Calories from Fat 33   Total Calories From: Fat 23% Protein 11% Carb. 66%

Vitamin A 7%   Vitamin C 34%   Iron 14%

Cabbage and Potato Soup

This delicious soup is very easy to make and is even better the second day. We enjoy it on a regular basis throughout the winter months.

8 SERVINGS

4 cups green cabbage, coarsely chopped

2 medium thin-skinned potatoes, unpeeled, cut into large chunks

1 medium onion, diced

2 ½ cups Garlic Stock (see page 80) or water

2 16-ounce cans stewed tomatoes

½ cup carrots, thinly sliced

3 tablespoons lemon juice

1 teaspoon sugar

1 teaspoon fresh thyme

1 teaspoon oregano

sea salt or salt substitute, to taste

freshly milled black pepper, to taste

chopped chives, for garnish

1. Combine onions, cabbage, and 2 cups of garlic stock or water in a large soup pot. Cook on medium heat for 15 minutes.

2. Add remaining ingredients. Bring to a boil, cover, reduce heat, and simmer for 1 hour, or until potatoes and cabbage are tender.

3. Serve garnished with fresh chopped chives.

Amount Per Serving

Calories 95   Calories from Fat 3   Total Calories From: Fat 3% Protein 10% Carb. 87%

Vitamin A 45%   Vitamin C 67%   Iron 7%

Kale and Lentil Soup

I first made this soup for its nutritional benefits, but continue to make it for the superior taste. If you don't have vegetable stock on hand, just add vegetable broth powder to the ingredients. You'll come back to this one time and time again.

8 SERVINGS

2 onions, diced

4 cloves garlic, minced

2 tablespoons water

1 tablespoon chili powder

1 teaspoon ground cumin

2 bay leaves

8 cups Basic Vegetable Stock
(see page 78)

¾ cup lentils, cleaned

2 cups tomatoes in purée, diced

1 pound kale, washed and chopped, with thick inner stalk removed

2 thin-skinned potatoes, unpeeled

2 tablespoons tamari soy sauce

1. Sauté onions and garlic in a large soup pot sprayed with olive oil cooking spray, stirring often, until onions are golden, about 8 minutes. Add a bit of water as needed to prevent burning. Add chili powder, cumin, and bay leaves; cook 1 minute more.

2. Add stock, lentils, and tomatoes. Bring to a boil. Cover and reduce heat. Simmer until lentils are just tender, about 25 minutes.

3. When lentils are tender, add kale and potatoes. Turn heat to high to resume a soft boil. Cover and reduce heat. Simmer until kale and potatoes are tender, about 15 minutes. Add soy sauce and serve.

Amount Per Serving

Calories 219   Calories from Fat 23   Total Calories From: Fat 10% Protein 16% Carb. 74%

Vitamin A 27%   Vitamin C 57%   Iron 22%

Cauliflower-Broccoli Bisque

You'll never miss the cream! The variations for this dish are endless. Substitute potatoes for the broccoli and you end up with a delicious cauliflower soup.

6 SERVINGS

extra-virgin olive oil cooking spray

1 small onion, diced

2 cloves garlic, minced

¾ pound broccoli florets

½ pound cauliflower florets

½ teaspoon sea salt or salt substitute

1 teaspoon white pepper

¼ teaspoon nutmeg

3 cups Basic Vegetable Stock (see page 78) or water

2 cups nonfat silken tofu

sprigs of parsley, for garnish

1. Spray a nonstick soup pot with olive oil cooking spray. Add onion and sauté over medium heat until golden brown. Add garlic and sauté for 2 minutes. Add water or vegetable stock as needed to prevent burning.

2. Add broccoli, cauliflower, salt, pepper, and nutmeg. Sauté until broccoli is bright green. Stir in vegetable stock and simmer, covered, until broccoli and cauliflower are tender.

3. Purée broccoli mixture with tofu until very creamy. Return to pot and warm through. Garnish with sprigs of parsley.

Amount Per Serving

Calories 128   Calories from Fat 13   Total Calories From: Fat 15% Protein 23% Carb. 62%

Vitamin A 21%   Vitamin C 140%   Iron 8%

Mixed Greens Stew

A delicious medley of mixed greens combines with beans and lots of garlic in this hearty dish. Serve with sourdough bread.

4 SERVINGS

2 bunches scallions, thinly sliced

4 cloves garlic, minced

1 tablespoon whole wheat flour

4 cups Basic Vegetable Stock (see page 78)

1 teaspoon tamari soy sauce

1 teaspoon white pepper

½ cup garbanzo beans, cooked

½ cup kidney beans, cooked

1 cup beet greens, chopped

1 cup kale, chopped

1 cup spinach, chopped

1 cup chard, chopped

1. In a large, heavy-bottomed soup pot sprayed with olive oil cooking spray, sauté scallions and garlic until scallions are soft, adding a bit of water as needed to prevent burning.

2. Stir in flour and cook for 2 to 3 minutes. Slowly add stock, soy sauce, and pepper. Cook until slightly thickened.

3. Add beans and greens. Simmer, stirring as needed to prevent burning, for 10 to 15 minutes, or until greens are tender.

Amount Per Serving

Calories 177   Calories from Fat 24   Total Calories From: Fat 13% Protein 20% Carb. 67%

Vitamin A 41%   Vitamin C 20%   Iron 24%

Sicilian Minestrone

Everyone who makes minestrone adds his or her own special touch. You could add or replace some of the vegetables listed here — turnips, spinach, or other greens are all good additions or substitutions. Be flexible and use what you have on hand.

6 SERVINGS

1 onion, finely diced

2 stalks celery, finely diced

4 carrots, finely diced

8 ounces new potatoes, quartered (unpeeled)

7 cups Basic Vegetable Stock (see page 78)

4 ounces pasta shells

2 zucchini, diced

2 cups cooked kidney beans

2 cups plum tomatoes, seeded and chopped

sea salt or salt substitute, to taste

freshly milled black pepper, to taste

1 tablespoon fresh basil, chopped, for garnish

1. Spray a large nonstick soup pot with olive oil cooking spray and sauté the onions until soft. Add the celery and carrots and cook 3 minutes longer.

2. Add the potatoes and vegetable stock and bring to a boil. Add the pasta shells and simmer for 10 minutes.

3. Add the zucchini and simmer for 10 minutes more. Add the beans, tomatoes, salt, and pepper and cook until heated through.

4. Serve garnished with chopped basil.

Amount Per Serving

Calories 276   Calories from Fat 32   Total Calories From: Fat 11% Protein 11% Carb. 78%

Vitamin A 295%   Vitamin C 83%   Iron 18%

Ratatouille

Ratatouille improves as it sits and is often better the next day when the flavors have mingled. Excellent served over brown rice or whole wheat pasta, or as a filling for crepes.

6 SERVINGS

2 onions, sliced

3 cloves garlic, minced

1 tablespoon fresh oregano, chopped

2 tablespoons fresh thyme, chopped

1 large eggplant,
unpeeled and cut into 1-inch cubes

1 sweet red pepper, cored, seeded,
and cut into ½-inch squares

1 green bell pepper, cored, seeded,
and cut into ½-inch squares

2 zucchini, sliced

8 tomatoes, cut into large chunks

3 stalks celery, sliced

3 carrots, thinly sliced

2 tablespoons cider vinegar

¼ cup unsalted sunflower seeds,
for garnish (optional)

1. Spray a large nonstick soup pot with olive oil cooking spray and sauté onions and garlic until lightly browned, adding a bit of water as needed to prevent burning.

2. Add herbs and stir for 30 seconds to release flavor from herbs.

3. Stir in vegetables and vinegar. Cover tightly and simmer over medium-low heat for 15-20 minutes.

4. Remove from heat and serve. Sprinkle sunflower seeds on top of each serving, if desired.

Amount Per Serving

Calories 245	Calories from Fat 43	Total Calories From: Fat 18% Protein 14% Carb. 68%	
		Vitamin A 242% Vitamin C 151% Iron 23%	

Gazpacho

This is one of our favorite summer soups, when fresh tomatoes are at their best.

8 SERVINGS

1 English cucumber, peeled and chopped medium fine

1 small onion, chopped medium fine

3 ripe tomatoes, chopped medium fine

½ sweet green pepper, diced medium fine

2 cloves garlic, finely minced

1 46-ounce can V-8 juice

½ cup cider vinegar

5 tablespoons fresh lemon juice

2 teaspoons green chili peppers, finely chopped

2 dashes Worcestershire sauce

2 dashes Tabasco pepper sauce

1 teaspoon tamari soy sauce

¼ teaspoon freshly milled black pepper

pinch of sugar

8 thin lemon slices, for garnish

Mix all ingredients together and chill for several hours or overnight. Garnish each serving with a thin lemon slice.

Amount Per Serving

Calories 18   Calories from Fat 1   Total Calories From: Fat 3% Protein 9% Carb. 88%

Vitamin A 1%   Vitamin C 18%   Iron 1%

Dressed-Up Stewed Tomatoes

Stewed tomatoes have always been one of my husband's favorite dishes. Adding the mushrooms and sherry simply makes it a gourmet delight.

6 SERVINGS

3 cups mushrooms, sliced

2 tablespoons cooking sherry

2 cloves garlic

2 teaspoons cornstarch

1 16-ounce can stewed tomatoes

sprig of parsley or chopped chives, for garnish

1. In a medium saucepan combine mushrooms, sherry, and garlic. Cook over medium heat, stirring frequently, 3 to 5 minutes, or until mushrooms are tender.

2. Dissolve cornstarch in 2 tablespoons water and add it to mushrooms along with tomatoes. Cook, stirring, until mixture comes to a boil. Boil 2 minutes, stirring constantly, until heated through.

3. Serve garnished with a sprig of parsley or finely chopped chives.

Amount Per Serving

Calories 60   Calories from Fat 2   Total Calories From: Fat 5% Protein 18% Carb. 77%

Vitamin A 21%   Vitamin C 47%   Iron 7%

Chilled Fresh Tomato Soup

This is a great soup for a hot summer day.

6 SERVINGS

1 medium onion, diced

6 cups fresh tomatoes, peeled and finely chopped

½ cup sweet green peppers, diced

1 cup Basic Vegetable Stock (see page 78)

¾ cup lemon juice

1 teaspoon cider vinegar

2 teaspoons sugar

1 tablespoon tamari soy sauce

1 tablespoon hot spicy salsa (optional)

freshly milled black pepper, to taste

cucumber rounds, for garnish

fat-free taco chips, for garnish (optional)

1. Sauté onions in a soup pot until softened, adding a bit of water as needed to prevent burning. Add tomatoes, green pepper, and vegetable stock to sautéed onions and bring to a boil. Lower heat and simmer, covered, 5 minutes.

2. Add remaining ingredients. Cover and simmer for an additional 10 minutes. Chill.

3. Place cucumber rounds on top of soup for garnish, or garnish with fat-free taco chips. Serve chilled.

Amount Per Serving

Calories 73   Calories from Fat 8   Total Calories From: Fat 12% Protein 10% Carb. 78%

Vitamin A 24%   Vitamin C 114%   Iron 6%

Centennial Garlic Soup

This aromatic, delicious soup is subtly flavored with the sweet taste of cooked garlic. Serve with crusty bread.

4 SERVINGS

20 cloves garlic, peeled and sliced

¼ cup onions, diced

2 tomatoes, peeled, seeded, and diced

½ cup carrots, sliced

¼ cup celery, sliced

4 cups Basic Vegetable Stock
(see page 78)

2 teaspoons cider vinegar

2 egg whites

1 teaspoon tamari soy sauce

freshly milled black pepper,
to taste

sea salt or salt substitute,
to taste

1. Heat a nonstick soup pot on medium heat. Spray with olive oil, add garlic, and sauté until very soft.* Add water as needed to prevent burning. Add the onion and continue stirring for 5 additional minutes.

2. Stir in the tomatoes and cook briefly. Add carrot, celery, and stock. Simmer, uncovered, until vegetables are cooked through. Add the vinegar and stir. Remove from heat.

3. Whisk egg white into soup mixture. Season to taste with salt and pepper. Reheat if necessary, but do not allow the soup to come to a boil.

*You can oven-roast the garlic if you prefer a sweeter flavor. See page 187 for instructions.

Amount Per Serving

Calories 100   Calories from Fat 20   Total Calories From: Fat 20% Protein 9% Carb. 71%

Vitamin A 93%   Vitamin C 48%   Iron 7%

Vegetarian Chili

Super-easy and super-quick to make, this chili is another one of our favorites.
I always keep the fixings in the pantry for a quick, delicious meal.

6 SERVINGS

extra-virgin olive oil cooking spray

1 cup onions, chopped

3 cloves garlic, minced

1 cup water

½ cup green bell peppers, diced

2 tablespoons chili powder

1½ teaspoons ground cumin

4 cups stewed tomatoes
(2 14-ounce cans)

2 cups kidney beans
(1 12-ounce can)

2 cups garbanzo beans
(1 12-ounce can)

red onion, finely chopped,
for garnish

1. Coat nonstick 4-quart soup pot with cooking spray; place over medium heat until hot. Add onion and garlic; sauté 5 minutes.

2. Add water and next 6 ingredients; bring to a boil. Reduce heat; simmer, uncovered for 30 minutes.

3. Ladle into individual soup bowls. Serve garnished with finely chopped red onion.

Amount Per Serving

Calories 364   Calories from Fat 30   Total Calories From: Fat 8% Protein 24% Carb. 68%

Vitamin A 30%   Vitamin C 76%   Iron 48%

White Bean Gumbo

A festive way to serve this dish is in individual "bowls," made by hollowing out French bread rolls.

6 SERVINGS

⅓ cup whole wheat flour

1-2 teaspoons water

3 ⅔ cups Basic Vegetable Stock (see page 78)

1 large onion, finely chopped

3 cloves garlic, minced

1 sweet green pepper, finely chopped

2 stalks celery, diced

2 cups tomatoes, chopped

½ cup fresh okra, sliced

1 teaspoon dried thyme

1 bay leaf

2 cups white navy beans, cooked and drained

½ teaspoon Red Chili Paste (see page 196) or more, to taste

3 cups brown rice, cooked

1. Place the flour in a nonstick skillet. Cook over medium-high heat, stirring constantly, until the flour is medium brown in color, about 7 minutes. Remove the skillet from the heat, and pour in ⅔ cup of the stock. Whisk until smooth.

2. Heat a heavy-bottomed 3-quart saucepan on medium-high heat. Sauté the onions in a teaspoon or two of water until soft. Add the garlic and sauté another minute.
Add the remaining stock and bring it to a boil. Whisk the flour mixture into the stock. Add the pepper, celery, tomatoes, okra, thyme, and bay leaf.

3. Bring to a boil, then reduce the heat to a simmer. Cover the pan loosely. Simmer the gumbo, stirring occasionally, for 15 minutes. Add the drained beans and Red Chili Paste.

4. Simmer until the vegetables are tender, about 15 minutes. Discard the bay leaf and serve over rice.

Amount Per Serving

Calories 420   Calories from Fat 9   Total Calories From: Fat 2% Protein 15% Carb. 83%

Vitamin A 10%   Vitamin C 54%   Iron 42%

Adzuki Bean-Butternut Squash Stew

Hearty and extremely nutritious, this stew is quick and easy to make. This is a great way to use leftover rice. It's also very good served over wild rice.

6 SERVINGS

½ cup Basic Vegetable Stock (see page 78)

1 tablespoon fresh ginger root, peeled, smashed, and minced

1 tablespoon tamari soy sauce

¼ teaspoon ground nutmeg

1 small butternut squash, peeled, seeds removed, and cut into small pieces

2 12-ounce cans adzuki beans, drained

sea salt or salt substitute, to taste

freshly milled black pepper, to taste

3 cups brown rice, cooked

1. Put vegetable stock, ginger root, soy sauce, and nutmeg into a large saucepan. Bring to a light simmer.

2. Add squash and cover. Cook for 10-15 minutes until squash is soft. Add beans and mix well, continuing to cook for another 2-3 minutes. Add salt and pepper if necessary. Add additional broth if stew becomes too dry.

3. Serve over brown rice.

Amount Per Serving

Calories 124   Calories from Fat 4   Total Calories From: Fat 3% Protein 8% Carb. 89%

Vitamin A 355%   Vitamin C 79%   Iron 9%

Black Bean Soup

Especially good on a cold winter day! I like to sprinkle freshly diced red onions or fat-free taco chips over the top just before serving, or put them on the table and let everyone add their own. Don't be afraid to double this recipe. It freezes beautifully!

6 SERVINGS

2 cups black beans, soaked overnight

2 teaspoons water or Basic Vegetable Stock for sautéing

1 medium onion, diced

3 cloves garlic, minced

⅓ cup celery, diced

¾ cup carrots, diced

1 cup sweet red peppers, diced

2 teaspoons ground sage

1 teaspoon fresh thyme

1 bay leaf

12 cups Basic Vegetable Stock (see page 78) or water

sea salt or salt substitute, to taste

1 small red onion, diced for topping (optional)

12 fat-free taco chips, broken into big chunks for topping (optional)

1. Drain and rinse the beans, discarding the soaking water.

2. In a large, heavy-bottomed soup pot, heat 2 teaspoons water and add the onion. Sauté the onion until it becomes translucent. Add the garlic, celery, carrots, red pepper, sage, thyme, and bay leaf. Sauté for several minutes. Add the drained beans and the vegetable broth. Bring to a boil and skim off any scum that may form on the top. Reduce heat and simmer for 2½ hours, stirring occasionally.

3. After 2½ hours, check the beans. They should be soft. Add salt and pepper (if desired, add 2 tablespoons powdered vegetable broth if you used water) to the beans. Continue cooking for 30 minutes.

4. Discard the bay leaf and purée about two-thirds of the soup. Return it to the pot. Adjust seasonings. Serve garnished with a little chopped onion and pieces of taco chips, if desired.

Amount Per Serving

Calories 258	Calories from Fat 37	Total Calories From: Fat 14% Protein 18% Carb. 68%
		Vitamin A 106% Vitamin C 61% Iron 22%

Joe's Special Sloppy Joes

This is just like you remember, only better. Serve with corn on the cob and cole slaw and have a feast.

6 SERVINGS

1 teaspoon extra-virgin olive oil

1 onion, diced

1 jalapeño pepper, finely diced

1 green pepper, diced

2 12-ounce packages veggie ground round or tempeh

⅔ cup catsup

1½ tablespoons Dijon mustard

1 tablespoon brown rice vinegar

1 teaspoon sea salt or salt substitute

¼ teaspoon freshly milled black pepper

6 whole grain burger buns, split

lettuce, for garnish (optional)

pickles, for garnish (optional)

sprouts, for garnish (optional)

1. In a large nonstick saucepan, heat the oil over medium heat and sauté the onion, stirring frequently to prevent sticking until onion is translucent, about 5 minutes. Add the peppers. Crumble the veggie ground round and add, continuing to cook for an additional 4 minutes, or until the veggie ground round browns.

2. Add the catsup, mustard, vinegar, salt, and pepper. Simmer for 20 minutes, stirring frequently.

3. Warm buns in oven if desired. Remove veggie mixture* from heat and spoon onto bottom half of each bun. Replace bun top and serve. Serve garnishes on the side.

* This mixture can be made ahead and frozen.

Amount Per Serving

Calories 67   Calories from Fat 12   Total Calories From: Fat 18% Protein 10% Carb. 72%

Vitamin A 13%   Vitamin C 33%   Iron 4%

Black Bean Burritos

For a gathering with friends or family with widely differing tastes, have a serve-yourself Mexican Feast! Cook the beans ahead (see variations), warm the tortillas in the oven, set out a variety of toppings, and serve buffet-style.

2 SERVINGS

½ cup cooked black beans

2 teaspoons salt-free
herb and spice blend*

⅛ teaspoon ground cumin

dash of ground red pepper

½ cup cooked long-grain rice

2 butter lettuce leaves**

2 fat-free whole wheat tortillas

¼ cup soy-style fat-free
Monterey Jack cheese, grated***

2 tablespoons green onion,
including tops, minced

2 tablespoons fat-free mild salsa

1. Combine first 4 ingredients in a small saucepan, stirring well. Cook over medium heat, stirring constantly, until thoroughly heated. Stir in cooked rice.

2. Place a lettuce leaf on each tortilla. Spoon bean mixture evenly down center of each tortilla. Top each with cheese, green onions, and salsa. Roll up tortillas and secure with wooden picks.

For variety, make up your own combinations using the following:

Beans: pinto, lentils, or adzuki

Veggies: shredded lettuce, scallion, green pepper, sprouts

Soy meat: veggie ground round***

Cheese: fat-free tofu cheese of choice***

On Top: Buffy's Eggless Mayonnaise (see page 195) or Home-Cooked Salsa
(see page 191)

*Prepared salt-free herb and spice blend can be found in the seasoning section of your health food store.

**Butter lettuce is sometimes known as bibb lettuce or Boston lettuce.

***Soy-style cheeses and veggie ground round can be found in your health food store.

Amount Per Serving

Calories 231	Calories from Fat 5	Total Calories From:	Fat 3%	Protein 12%	Carb. 85%
		Vitamin A 1%	Vitamin C 2%	Iron 18%	

Tummy-Tempting
Tempeh-Mushroom Scramble

This hearty sandwich filling can be served buffet-style with crackers or crudités.

6 SERVINGS

extra-virgin olive oil cooking spray

1 medium onion, diced

2 cloves garlic, minced

½ pound mushrooms, thinly sliced*

½ green bell pepper, diced

1 small chili pepper, minced

8 ounces tempeh or ground
vegetable meat, crumbled

1 28-ounce can crushed tomatoes

1 tablespoon honey

1 tablespoon Worcestershire sauce

2 tablespoons apple cider vinegar

sea salt or salt substitute, to taste**

freshly milled black pepper, to taste**

6 hamburger buns

1. In a nonstick skillet that has been sprayed with olive oil cooking spray, sauté onions over medium heat for 5 minutes or until they are soft.

2. Add garlic, mushrooms, peppers, and crumbled tempeh. Cook until vegetables are softened, about 7 minutes.

3. Add tomatoes. When heated through, stir in honey, Worcestershire sauce, vinegar, and additional salt and pepper if necessary. Make sure to taste along the way, adjusting the condiments to suit your preference for salty, sweet, or sour flavors. Serve hot on hamburger buns.

*We like portabella mushrooms in this dish, but you can use other mushrooms as well.

** You can substitute soy sauce for salt and pepper if you wish.

Amount Per Serving

Calories 154	Calories from Fat 32	Total Calories From: Fat 20% Protein 26% Carb. 54%
Vitamin A 22%	Vitamin C 72%	Iron 12%

Chili-Lentil Pockets

Perfect for cool autumn outings.

4 SERVINGS

1 quart water

1 cup lentils, rinsed and sorted, discarding any debris

1 bay leaf

2 small dried chili peppers

¾ teaspoon cumin

2 cloves garlic, finely minced

1 tablespoon extra-virgin olive oil

3 tablespoons balsamic vinegar

½ cup green onions, including tops, thinly sliced

1 cup celery, cut into 2-inch matchsticks

¼ cup red bell peppers, cut into 2-inch matchsticks

4 whole wheat pita pockets (6-inch diameter), cut in half

Buffy's Eggless Mayonnaise (see page 195) or your favorite fat-free sandwich dressing

1. Place water, lentils, bay leaf, chili peppers, and cumin in a 4-quart pan and bring to a boil. Reduce heat, cover, and simmer until lentils are tender (approximately 40 minutes). Drain lentils, discarding chili peppers and bay leaf, and let cool.

2. Combine garlic, olive oil, and vinegar in a large bowl. Add lentils and gently mix.

3. Up to 3 hours before serving, add onions, celery, and bell pepper to lentil mixture; stir well. Scoop into pita halves and top with Buffy's Eggless Mayonnaise, or a fat-free version from your favorite health food store.

Amount Per Serving

Calories 223   Calories from Fat 41   Total Calories From: Fat 18% Protein 26% Carb. 56%

Vitamin A 10%   Vitamin C 33%   Iron 29%

Chickpea Sandwich Salad

This can be used as an appetizer, side dish, dip, or sandwich salad. Try it in pita bread with fresh greens and grated carrots, on crackers, or with vegetable crudités.

6 SERVINGS

4 cups cooked chickpeas

½ cup celery, coarsely chopped

½ cup onions, finely chopped

2 tablespoons fresh lemon juice

½ cup Buffy's Eggless Mayonnaise (see page 195)

1 tablespoon dried powdered kelp*

sea salt, to taste

freshly milled black pepper, to taste

6 whole wheat fat-free pita pockets, cut in half

2 tomatoes, chopped

2 cups salad lettuce or sprouts of your choice

1. Place the chickpeas in a food processor and process until coarsely chopped. Transfer to a bowl.

2. Add the rest of the ingredients and mix.

3. Serve stuffed into pita pockets with chopped tomatoes and lettuce or sprouts.

*Dried powdered kelp can be found in most good health food stores.

Amount Per Serving

Calories 508   Calories from Fat 73   Total Calories From: Fat 14% Protein 20% Carb. 66%

Vitamin A 2%   Vitamin C 15%   Iron 47%

Buffy's Hearty Luncheon Salad

Served with soup and a baguette, this salad becomes the center of a hearty meal.

6 SERVINGS

8 ounces spinach

6 ounces arugula

1 head butter lettuce
(or substitute your favorite salad lettuce)

1 cup red cabbage, chopped

1 Granny Smith apple,
cut in bite-size pieces

⅓ cup raisins

½ cup toasted pumpkin seeds

4 green onions, including tops,
finely sliced

8 cherry tomatoes, cut in half

1 cup broccoli sprouts

½ cup chickpeas, cooked

Orange-Soy Dressing (see page 194)

1. Wash spinach, arugula, and butter lettuce. Drain and spin or pat dry. Tear greens into bite-sized pieces and place in a large salad bowl.

2. Add all other salad ingredients. Set aside.

3. Make Orange-Soy Dressing (see page 194) or use your favorite fat-free dressing. Add to salad before serving.

Amount Per Serving

Calories 122	Calories from Fat 11	Total Calories From: Fat 9% Protein 14% Carb. 77%
		Vitamin A 21% Vitamin C 28% Iron 11%

Pear Salad with Miso-Tamarind Sauce

Tamarind can be difficult to find, so ask your health food store to order it for you if you can't find it on the shelf, or order from one of the sources in the back of this book. This salad is well worth the effort. It's a great special treat for guests, too!

4 SERVINGS

1 teaspoon red or barley miso

1 teaspoon tamarind concentrate (see glossary)

2 teaspoons maple syrup

1 teaspoon arrowroot

3 cloves garlic, finely minced

2 tablespoons ginger root, finely minced

2 pears, seeded and sliced into 8 sections each

⅓ cup + 1 tablespoon water

1 tablespoon tomato paste concentrate

1 teaspoon sea salt or salt substitute

1 head butter lettuce* or salad greens of your choice, to serve four

toasted almonds, for garnish (optional)

1. Combine miso, tamarind, maple syrup, arrowroot, garlic, ginger root, and 1 tablespoon water in a bowl and stir until smooth. Set aside.

2. Over medium-high heat, sauté pears in a nonstick skillet until lightly browned, about 5-7 minutes. Remove with a slotted spoon and arrange over salad greens.

3. Return pan to heat and add miso sauce, ⅓ cup water, and salt. Turn heat to medium-high and stir in tomato paste. When sauce thickens, remove from heat and drizzle over salad.

*Butter lettuce is sometimes referred to as bibb or Boston lettuce.

Amount Per Serving

Calories 74   Calories from Fat 3   Total Calories From: Fat 5% Protein 3% Carb. 92%

Vitamin A 2%   Vitamin C 9%   Iron 2%

Fruit and Berry Salad

For this dish, the fruits should be kept separate until serving time so each retains its unique character. This can be either served as a luncheon salad or as a dessert.

6 SERVINGS

1 navel orange,
peeled and segments
removed from membrane

3 very ripe kiwis,
peeled and cut into eight rounds

1 cup very ripe pineapple, cubed

1 cup fresh raspberries, cleaned

1 cup fresh blackberries, cleaned

1 cup fresh strawberries, cleaned and
halved, with stems removed

Sauce:

3 tablespoons apricot preserves

1 tablespoon fructose

1½ teaspoons fresh orange juice

¾ cup water

1½ teaspoons fresh lemon juice

⅛ teaspoon zest of fresh organic lemon

1teaspoon vanilla extract

1. Prepare fruit, keeping each kind of fruit separate. Refrigerate until ready to use.

2. While fruit is chilling, prepare the sauce. Combine apricot preserves, fructose, orange juice, and ¾ cup water in a 1-quart saucepan. Bring to a boil over medium-high heat. Reduce heat and simmer gently for 4-5 minutes. Remove from heat.

3. Stir in lemon juice, lemon zest, and vanilla extract. Stir to blend. Set sauce aside to cool to room temperature.

4. Remove fruit from refrigerator and divide it equally among 6 serving plates. Drizzle a tablespoon of sauce over each plate of fruit.

Amount Per Serving

Calories 123	Calories from Fat 6	Total Calories From: Fat 4% Protein 4% Carb. 92%
		Vitamin A 4% Vitamin C 131% Iron 4%

Apple-Quinoa Salad

The diversity of flavors, colors, and textures of the ingredients in this dish will captivate the most jaded gourmet.

8 SERVINGS

1 cup Basic Quinoa (see page 74)

⅓ cup cider vinegar

3 tablespoons apple juice concentrate

¼ teaspoon ground allspice

¼ teaspoon pepper

1 clove garlic, minced

1 red delicious apple,
cored and cut into ½-inch cubes

½ cup carrots, shredded

⅓ cup red onions, diced

⅓ cup jicama, thinly sliced
(see glossary)

¼ cup fresh mint leaves, chopped

butter lettuce leaves,* rinsed

sea salt or salt substitute, to taste

1. Pour quinoa into a fine strainer and rinse well under cool running water.

2. In a 1½ to 2-quart pan, combine quinoa and 2 cups water. Bring to a boil on high heat, then turn heat to low, cover, and simmer until grain is tender to bite, 10 to 15 minutes. Let cool.

3. Combine vinegar, apple juice concentrate, allspice, pepper, and garlic. Mix with cool quinoa.

4. Mix apple cubes, carrot, onion, jicama, and mint leaves with quinoa.

5. Mound salad on a lettuce-lined platter. Add salt to taste.

*Butter lettuce is also known as bibb or Boston lettuce.

Amount Per Serving

Calories 111   Calories from Fat 13   Total Calories From: Fat 11% Protein 12% Carb. 77%

Vitamin A 41%   Vitamin C 13%   Iron 13%

Buffy's Favorite Tofu Salad

I made this salad for a friend from Hong Kong, and she asked for the recipe. I was delighted, since she had taught me the basics of cooking with tofu.

4 SERVINGS

3 cloves garlic, finely minced

2 teaspoons ginger root, peeled and grated

1 teaspoon capers

1 teaspoon Red Chili Paste (see page 196), or more if you like it hot

2 tablespoons tamari soy sauce

1½ tablespoons rice vinegar

1 teaspoon dark sesame oil

1 12-ounce cake low-fat tofu, pressed firmly

½ cup green onions, finely chopped

½ cup sweet red or green bell peppers, finely diced

2 tablespoons fresh parsley, chopped

1. Combine the garlic, ginger root, capers, Red Chili Paste, soy sauce, rice vinegar, and sesame oil in a small bowl and whisk until blended. Set aside.

2. Crumble the tofu into a separate bowl. Add the remaining ingredients and combine with the garlic-ginger mix. Serve or chill until later.

Amount Per Serving

Calories 43   Calories from Fat 11   Total Calories From: Fat 26% Protein 16% Carb. 58%

Vitamin A 66%   Vitamin C 138%   Iron 5%

Three-Bean Pasta Salad

Whenever we take a trip I make this salad along with some crudités, and we have a great snack while we're traveling. Sometimes I blanch broccoli, cauliflower, and carrots and add them to this recipe. It makes a very colorful dish and adds extra texture, as well as nutrition.

6 SERVINGS

2 ounces bow tie pasta, uncooked

1 12-ounce can cut green beans, drained

1 12-ounce can garbanzo beans, drained

1 12-ounce can kidney beans, drained

1 cup sweet green pepper, chopped

1 cup sweet red pepper, chopped

½ cup cider vinegar

1 tablespoon sugar

1 teaspoon garlic, minced

¼ teaspoon sea salt

¼ teaspoon freshly milled black pepper

1. Cook pasta according to package directions, omitting salt and fat. Drain; rinse with cold water, and drain again. Combine cooked pasta, green beans, and next 4 ingredients in a bowl; toss well.

2. Combine vinegar and remaining ingredients in a small bowl, stirring well. Pour vinegar mixture over pasta mixture. Toss well.

3. Cover and chill for at least 2 hours. Toss gently before serving.

Amount Per Serving

Calories 77	Calories from Fat 5	Total Calories From: Fat 7% Protein 11% Carb. 82%
Vitamin A 16%	Vitamin C 59%	Iron 5%

Mediterranean Lentil Salad

Don't let the long list of ingredients scare you. This is a simple dish to make and one of our favorites.

6 SERVINGS

4 cups water

1 cup lentils, washed and drained

1 teaspoon fresh thyme

3 cloves garlic

2 bay leaves

⅓ cup sun-dried tomatoes

½ cup celery or bok choy

¼ cup red onions, diced

½ cup fresh parsley, chopped

½ cup yellow, orange,
or red sweet peppers, diced

½ teaspoon capers (optional)

Dressing:

2 tablespoons extra-virgin olive oil

3 tablespoons balsamic vinegar

1 teaspoon ground fennel

1 teaspoon Dijon mustard

sea salt or salt substitute, to taste

freshly milled black pepper, to taste

1. In a medium saucepan, add the water, lentils, thyme, garlic, and bay leaves and bring them to a boil. Reduce heat and simmer for 20 minutes, stirring occasionally.

2. While the lentils simmer, cover the sun-dried tomatoes with boiling water and set aside.

3. Combine celery, onions, parsley, peppers, and capers (if using) in a large bowl.

4. In a separate bowl, whisk the dressing ingredients until smooth.

5. When the sun-dried tomatoes have softened, drain and mince them. Add them to the vegetables.

6. Drain the lentils and discard the bay leaves. Remove the garlic, mash it, and mix it back into the lentils. Toss the lentils with the vegetables and add dressing.

Amount Per Serving

Calories 155   Calories from Fat 25   Total Calories From: Fat 16% Protein 26% Carb. 58%

Vitamin A 19%   Vitamin C 45%   Iron 20%

Garden Vegetable Couscous Salad

The garlic lemon vinaigrette in this delicious dish enlivens the assortment of colorful vegetables. This also works well if you substitute the couscous with quinoa.

6 SERVINGS

2½ cups cooked couscous

½ cup carrots,
cut into bite-size pieces

½ small red bell pepper,
stem and seeds removed,
cut into bite-size pieces

½ small green bell pepper,
stem and seeds removed,
cut into bite-size pieces

½ cup celery,
cut into bite-size pieces

4 green onions,
white and light-green parts only

12 cherry tomatoes, halved

1 tablespoon extra-virgin olive oil

1 tablespoon lemon juice

2 cloves garlic, minced

sea salt, to taste

freshly milled black pepper to taste

lemon zest, for garnish

1. Blanch the carrots, bell peppers, and celery in boiling water until just tender. Drain well. Transfer them to a serving bowl. Thinly slice the green onions crosswise and add to peppers. Add cherry tomatoes.

2. In a small bowl, whisk together the olive oil, lemon juice, and garlic. Season with salt and pepper. Drizzle over vegetables and toss. Garnish with lemon zest.

3. Spoon vegetables and sauce over couscous in individual bowls.

Amount Per Serving

Calories 304   Calories from Fat 25   Total Calories From: Fat 8% Protein 13% Carb. 79%

Vitamin A 6%   Vitamin C 19%   Iron 5%

Cold Leeks with Tomato Sauce

A perfect appetizer salad. This dish is the very essence of spring.

6 SERVINGS

3 to 4 large ripe tomatoes

2 cloves garlic, minced

3 green onions, finely chopped

2 tablespoons parsley, minced

2 to 3 tablespoons fresh basil

1 bay leaf

1 tablespoon fresh thyme

sea salt or salt substitute, to taste

freshly milled black pepper, to taste

2 carrots, peeled and sliced

1 celery stalk, sliced

6 leeks, trimmed, halved, and rinsed

chives, for garnish

1. Immerse tomatoes in boiling water for about 30 seconds, or until skins begin to loosen. Peel, quarter, and set aside.

2. Heat a large nonstick skillet over low heat. Spray with olive oil cooking spray.
Add garlic, scallions, and parsley and cook 1 minute. Add tomatoes, basil, bay leaf, thyme, salt, and pepper. Cover and cook 5 minutes. Remove cover. Increase heat and cook sauce, stirring constantly until thickened. Remove from heat and set aside.

3. Bring 3 quarts water to a simmer in a deep skillet or Dutch oven with 2 teaspoons sea salt, bouquet garni, carrots, and celery. Slip the leeks into the pan and cook gently until tender when pierced with a knife, 15 to 25 minutes. Lift them out and arrange them, cut side up, on a platter. (Save the cooking liquid for an excellent broth for soup.)

4. Spoon tomato sauce over leeks and garnish with snips of chives.

Amount Per Serving

Calories 101	Calories from Fat 6	Total Calories From: Fat 5% Protein 10% Carb. 85%
		Vitamin A 12% Vitamin C 54% Iron 19%

Spinach Salad with Berries

We first had this delicious salad while on a picnic with friends. It was a potluck, so we all brought our favorites. This is what Kathy brought. It was a real hit. She scattered nuts over the top, but I have left them off to keep the fat at a minimum.

4 SERVINGS

6 ounces fresh spinach

1 cup fresh strawberries or raspberries

½ small red onion, thinly sliced

Dressing:

1 tablespoon extra-virgin olive oil

2 tablespoons balsamic vinegar

2 tablespoons rice vinegar

1 tablespoon maple syrup

2 teaspoons Dijon mustard

sea salt or salt substitute, to taste

freshly milled black pepper, to taste

1. Wash spinach and pat or spin dry. Add red onions. Set aside.

2. Whisk the dressing ingredients until smooth.

3. Pour dressing over spinach mixture, toss salad, and add the berries in a decorative manner.

Amount Per Serving

Calories 60   Calories from Fat 5   Total Calories From: Fat 8% Protein 13% Carb. 79%

Vitamin A 58%   Vitamin C 36%   Iron 8%

Radish and Orange Salad

A refreshing, relish-type salad that is quick and easy to make. It's great on a hot summer day.

6 SERVINGS

2 bunches long or round red radishes

2 tablespoons fresh lemon juice

2 tablespoons orange juice

sea salt or salt substitute,
to taste

2 navel oranges,
peeled and sectioned, with seeds,
pith, and membrane removed

cinnamon, to taste

mint leaves, for garnish

1. Wash, trim, and grate radishes. Place grated radishes in double-thickness cheese cloth and squeeze out all excess liquid. Place in serving dish.

2. Blend lemon and orange juice together. Sprinkle over grated radishes and add salt to taste. Toss lightly to blend. Chill.

3. Just before serving, mix in oranges and dust very lightly with cinnamon. Garnish with mint leaves.

Amount Per Serving

Calories 26	Calories from Fat 0	Total Calories From: Fat 2% Protein 8% Carb. 90%
		Vitamin A 2% Vitamin C 49% Iron 0%

Not Your Plain Old Broccoli Salad

This is a great side dish, but if you wish to turn it into an easy, quick main dish, just add pasta. Serve with a tossed salad on the side and you have a cool, refreshing meal.

4 SERVINGS

½ teaspoon extra-virgin olive oil

2 ½ teaspoons tamari soy sauce

2 tablespoons fresh lemon juice

2 tablespoons seasoned
rice wine vinegar

2 teaspoons ginger root,
peeled and grated

zest of one lemon

1 teaspoon freshly milled black pepper

1 clove garlic, minced

4 cups broccoli florets,
steamed to crisp-tender

⅓ cup green onion,
cut in thin diagonal slivers

2 tablespoons slivered almonds
(optional)

1. To make the dressing, whisk together the oil, soy sauce, lemon juice, vinegar, ginger root, lemon zest, pepper, and garlic.

2. Toss broccoli and scallions with dressing.

3. Serve on a bed of lettuce. Sprinkle with slivered almonds for added crunch, if desired.

Amount Per Serving

Calories 49   Calories from Fat 8   Total Calories From: Fat 17% Protein 26% Carb. 57%

Vitamin A 28%   Vitamin C 146%   Iron 6%

Hawaiian Cole Slaw

Prepare this slaw a day in advance so it has time to develop some depth.

8 SERVINGS

4 cups cabbage, finely shredded

½ cup carrots, finely shredded

¼ cup sweet green peppers, very finely chopped

1 12-ounce can unsweetened crushed pineapple

2 tablespoons Buffy's Eggless Mayonnaise (see page 195)

1 tablespoon brown rice vinegar

1 teaspoon Dijon mustard

1 tablespoon brown sugar

sea salt or salt substitute, to taste

freshly milled black pepper, to taste

1. In a large bowl, combine first 4 ingredients.

2. In a small bowl, combine remaining ingredients. Add to cabbage mixture, mixing well.

3. Chill. Mix before serving.

Amount Per Serving

Calories 32   Calories from Fat 2   Total Calories From: Fat 6% Protein 8% Carb. 86%

Vitamin A 40%   Vitamin C 380%   Iron 2%

Cool Cabbage Salad

This is a delicious, low-fat, sweet and sour salad with a pleasant bite. Take it along on a picnic.

8 SERVINGS

5 cups red cabbage, grated

5 cups green cabbage, grated

2 tablespoons rice vinegar

½ cup raisins

1 tablespoon extra-virgin olive oil

2 tablespoons honey

½ teaspoon black pepper, coarsely grated

1 teaspoon celery seeds

½ teaspoon sea salt or salt substitute

1. Combine cabbages and set aside.

2. Combine remaining ingredients and mix them with the cabbage.

3. Chill thoroughly (1 hour or longer) allowing enough time for the flavors to blend, then serve.

Amount Per Serving

Calories 84   Calories from Fat 9   Total Calories From: Fat 10% Protein 7% Carb. 83%

Vitamin A 1%   Vitamin C 77%   Iron 5%

Cabbage-Tofu Salad

This is a super-simple, tasty salad with a beautiful presentation. However, do toss the salad before eating.

8 SERVINGS

1 pound soft tofu

4 cups Napa cabbage, finely shredded

2 cups spinach leaves, finely shredded

1 cup red cabbage, finely shredded

1 jicama, cut into 2-inch matchsticks

1 carrot, shaved into thin curls
with a vegetable peeler

5 radishes, cut into 2-inch matchsticks

freshly milled black pepper, to taste

sea salt or salt substitute, to taste

1 tablespoon black sesame seeds,
for garnish

fat-free dressing

1. Bring a medium saucepan of water to a gentle simmer. Dice the tofu and gently slide it into the water. Simmer over moderate heat for 2 minutes, then transfer to paper towels to drain.

2. Arrange the tofu and vegetables on a large platter in a geometric pattern, separating each ingredient. Sprinkle the black sesame seeds over the soft tofu. Season with salt and pepper.

3. Serve your favorite fat-free dressing on the side. Let each guest blend his or her own salad.

Amount Per Serving

Calories 112	Calories from Fat 32	Total Calories From: Fat 29%	Protein 25%	Carb. 46%
		Vitamin A 72%	Vitamin C 63%	Iron 25%

Southwest Rice and Bean Salad

Lovers of spicy food will adore this salad. Serve it over a bed of lettuce, add some fat-free taco chips, and you have an easy lunch with a Mexican flair.

6 SERVINGS

1 16-ounce can black beans, rinsed and drained

1 cup cooked long-grain brown rice

1 sweet onion, diced

1 clove garlic, crushed and minced

1 sweet green pepper, seeded and diced

1 sweet red pepper, seeded and diced

2 red chili peppers, cored, seeded and finely chopped

4 large tomatoes, cut into cubes

4 ounces low-fat silken tofu

sea salt or salt substitute, to taste

freshly milled black pepper, to taste

½ teaspoon chili powder, or to taste

¼ teaspoon ground cumin

½ teaspoon dried oregano

1. In a large bowl, combine beans, rice, onion, garlic, peppers, and tomatoes. Mix well.

2. In a blender combine the tofu and spices. Add to the bean and rice mixture, mixing until well blended.

3. Chill several hours to blend flavors. Stir before serving.

Amount Per Serving

Calories 123   Calories from Fat 11   Total Calories From: Fat 9% Protein 18% Carb. 73%

Vitamin A 67%   Vitamin C 180%   Iron 11%

Chili Bean Salad

A delicious combination of Southwestern flavors, perfect for a potluck, lunchbox entrée, or a summer meal.

4 SERVINGS

2 cups kidney beans, cooked

⅔ cup red onions, finely chopped

¾ cup sweet green peppers, finely chopped

¼ cup plain nonfat soy yogurt or low-fat silken tofu

1 teaspoon chili powder

¼ teaspoon ground cumin

¼ teaspoon dried oregano

½ teaspoon sea salt or salt substitute

1 head of salad lettuce of your choice

1. In a large bowl, combine kidney beans, onions, and green pepper. Mix well.

2. In a small bowl, combine yogurt or tofu and spices. Add to bean mixture, mixing well.

3. Chill. Serve over a bed of lettuce.

Amount Per Serving

Calories 331   Calories from Fat 4   Total Calories From: Fat 1% Protein 28% Carb. 71%

Vitamin A 6%   Vitamin C 38%   Iron 50%

Cancún Taco Salad

A great south-of-the-border salad! You can also stuff the mixture into fat-free taco shells and top with your favorite fixings.

2 SERVINGS

1 pound tempeh

3 tablespoons tamari soy sauce

¼ cup lime juice, fresh-squeezed

1 tablespoon chili powder

extra-virgin olive oil cooking spray

1 onion, chopped

¼ cup cilantro, chopped

shredded lettuce

1. Chop tempeh into small pieces and place in a mixing bowl. Combine tamari, lime juice, and chili powder in small bowl. Pour over the tempeh. Let stand 30 minutes. The longer it sits, the better the absorption of the flavor.

2. Spray a nonstick skillet or wok with extra-virgin olive oil cooking spray and sauté the onion over medium heat about 5 minutes, or until soft. Add marinated tempeh and keep mixture moving in the skillet until tempeh turns golden brown. Add cilantro just before serving.

3. Serve over a bed of lettuce.

Amount Per Serving

Calories 81   Calories from Fat 8   Total Calories From: Fat 9% Protein 14% Carb. 77%

Vitamin A 36%   Vitamin C 149%   Iron 8%

Black-Eyed Peas Salad

Aromatic and tangy, serve this on a bed of greens and garnish with mint sprigs. This salad can also be used to make a wrap, or stuff it into pita bread.

4 SERVINGS

2 tablespoons rice wine vinegar

1 teaspoon Dijon mustard

1 teaspoon extra-virgin olive oil

1 clove garlic, minced

¼ teaspoon dried oregano

¼ teaspoon dried basil

⅛ teaspoon nutmeg, grated

2 cups spinach, shredded

1½ cups cooked black-eyed peas

2 plum tomatoes, chopped

1 small onion, thinly sliced

salad greens of choice

1. To make the dressing, whisk together the vinegar, mustard, and oil. Stir in the garlic, oregano, basil, and nutmeg.

2. In a large bowl, combine the spinach, peas, tomatoes, and onion. Pour on the dressing and toss well to combine.

3. Serve on a bed of salad greens.

Amount Per Serving

Calories 99	Calories from Fat 17	Total Calories From: Fat 17% Protein 20% Carb. 63%
		Vitamin A 43% Vitamin C 32% Iron 12%

Main Dishes

▼

Main dishes are the centerpieces of your meals, or the theme that determines the foods you want to serve. Some are hearty enough to serve by themselves or with bread, while others welcome the company of vegetable side dishes, soups, and salads. Many of the recipes that follow take less than an hour to prepare. There is something for everyone's taste, from mild to spicy, from egg fu-yung to Tuscan beans. Best of all, they look inviting and taste great!

Cook Extra Portions

When you cook grains, dried beans, long-cooking vegetables, or vegetable soups, consider cooking enough for two or more meals. In most cases, this involves little or no extra work, and that extra cooked rice or beans will come in handy for a later menu when you don't have the time to prepare a full meal or don't feel like cooking. Spoon the extra portions into containers that can go from the freezer to the microwave. These foods freeze and reheat beautifully.

Algerian Curried Couscous

Couscous can be used as a base grain for beans and stews, as well as making a nice salad when fresh vegetables and a dressing are added to the cooked grain. It's a great dish to take on those outings or picnics.

6 SERVINGS

2 ½ cups Basic Vegetable Stock (see page 78)

¾ cup golden raisins

6 tablespoons lemon juice

3 tablespoons crystallized ginger, finely chopped

2 teaspoons extra-virgin olive oil

¾ teaspoon curry powder

sea salt or salt substitute, to taste

freshly milled black pepper, to taste

1 ½ cups couscous

½ cup celery, thinly sliced

⅓ cup green onions, including tops, thinly sliced

3 tablespoons cilantro, chopped

¼ cup almonds, coarsely chopped (optional)

4 sprigs of parsley, for garnish

1. Bring broth to a boil over high heat. Stir in raisins, lemon juice, ginger, olive oil, curry powder, salt, pepper, and couscous. Cover pan and remove from heat. Let stand for 5 to 10 minutes. Fluff couscous with a fork. (At this point, you may cover and refrigerate until next day; bring to room temperature before serving.)

2. Serve couscous warm or at room temperature. Just before serving, stir in celery, onions, and chopped cilantro. Mound couscous mixture in a serving dish. Sprinkle with almonds if used, and garnish with sprigs of parsley.

Amount Per Serving

Calories 285   Calories from Fat 26   Total Calories From: Fat 9% Protein 10% Carb. 81%

Vitamin A 3%   Vitamin C 16%   Iron 9%

Bombay Dhal

A spicy mélange of flavors, dhal is great topped with your favorite tomato sauce. It can be frozen up to two months. Thaw at room temperature for 3-4 hours, and then gently reheat on top of the stove.

4 SERVINGS

extra-virgin olive oil cooking spray

½ pound yellow split peas, soaked overnight and drained

1 large onion, peeled and diced

2 cloves garlic, finely chopped

2½ teaspoons ground cumin

1¼ teaspoons ground turmeric

2 green onions, thinly sliced

2½ teaspoons lemon juice

sea salt or salt substitute, to taste

freshly milled black pepper, to taste

1½ tablespoons fresh parsley, chopped

tomato sauce

1. Cook the split peas in boiling, unsalted water for 30–40 minutes, or until they are tender. Drain thoroughly.

2. Heat a nonstick skillet sprayed with olive oil cooking spray. Add onion and cook for 3 minutes, stirring frequently. Add garlic and cook for 1 minute longer. Stir in the cumin and turmeric and cook for 3 minutes. Add water if needed to prevent burning.

3. Stir in the split peas, green onions, and lemon juice. Season with salt and pepper. Cook for an additional 2–3 minutes, then taste and adjust the seasoning if necessary.

4. Turn the mixture onto a heated serving dish. Sprinkle with chopped parsley. Serve hot with tomato sauce on the side.

Amount Per Serving

Calories 43	Calories from Fat 4	Total Calories From: Fat 10%	Protein 12%	Carb. 78%

Vitamin A 0%   Vitamin C 12%   Iron 7%

Quinoa with Currants

This unique whole grain, which was the staple food of the Incas, is also rich in calcium and iron. I use a boiling method, similar to cooking pasta, for cooking this grain.

6 SERVINGS

¾ cup rinsed quinoa*

1½ cup water

½ teaspoon sea salt
or salt substitute

1 red onion, finely diced

½ teaspoon ground cumin

¼ teaspoon ground cinnamon

¼ teaspoon ground coriander

¼ teaspoon ground ginger

⅛ teaspoon turmeric

¼ teaspoon freshly milled
black pepper

¼ cup cilantro, chopped

¼ cup currants

1 teaspoon grated orange
or lemon zest

1. Rinse quinoa with warm water and drain through a fine strainer.

2. Bring 1½ cups water with ¼ teaspoon sea salt added to a boil. Add the quinoa. Cover and reduce heat. Simmer for 15 minutes.

3. Meanwhile, heat a nonstick skillet. Add the onion, spices, and black pepper. Cook gently until softened, about 10 minutes. Add a bit of water if needed to prevent burning. Season with remaining sea salt.

4. Drain the quinoa when it's done and toss with the onion mixture along with the cilantro, currants, and orange or lemon zest. Serve hot or at room temperature.

*Quinoa can be found in most good health food stores.

Amount Per Serving

Calories 103   Calories from Fat 12   Total Calories From: Fat 12% Protein 13% Carb. 75%

Vitamin A 1%   Vitamin C 20%   Iron 13%

Wheat-Berry Sauté

Wheat berries provide a "chewiness" in this tasty dish. For special occasions, sprinkle a small amount of toasted almond slivers over the top. Start this dish the night before you wish to serve it.

4 SERVINGS

4 cups water

¾ cup wheat berries*

extra-virgin olive oil cooking spray

1 onion, diced

2 cloves garlic, minced

1 cup tomatoes, diced

½ cup dried apricots, diced

½ cup water

⅓ cup (packed) fresh basil leaves, chopped

½ teaspoon freshly milled black pepper

sea salt or salt substitute, to taste (optional)

toasted almond slivers (optional)

1. Soak the wheat berries in ample water to cover in a medium covered saucepan for at least 8 hours.

2. Drain the soaked wheat berries, using a colander or a large sieve. Return them to the saucepan with the water and bring to boil, then reduce heat to low, cover, and simmer 45 minutes, or to desired tenderness. Drain well.

3. Spray a large nonstick skillet with extra-virgin olive oil spray. Add onion and cook over medium-high heat, stirring frequently, until wilted, 4 to 5 minutes. Add garlic and cook 2 more minutes.

4. Add tomato and apricots. Stir gently. Add water and cook until absorbed, 3 to 4 minutes. Remove from heat. Let cool. Toss with basil, pepper, and salt (if used). Garnish with toasted almond slivers, if desired, and serve chilled or at room temperature.

*You will find wheat berries in most good health food stores.

Amount Per Serving

Calories 101   Calories from Fat 15   Total Calories From: Fat 15% Protein 7% Carb. 78%

Vitamin A 44%   Vitamin C 29%   Iron 9%

Vegetable Paella

Paella, a traditional Spanish dish, was originally cooked on an open fire in a large flat pan called a paellera. A paella may include a variety of meats, vegetables, and seafood, and each region of Spain has its own version. In this vegetarian version, we use seasoned seitan in place of meats or seafood for a delicious medley of flavors.

8 SERVINGS

extra-virgin olive oil cooking spray

1 large onion, diced

3 cloves garlic, minced or pressed

1 cup celery, finely chopped

¼ teaspoon saffron threads

1 tablespoon fresh thyme

1 sweet red pepper, thinly sliced

1 cup asparagus,
cut into 1-inch pieces

1 cup fresh or frozen green peas

2 zucchini, thinly sliced

4 Italian tomatoes, thinly sliced

¼ pound chicken-flavored seitan,
cut into strips (see glossary)

sea salt or salt substitute, to taste

freshly milled black pepper, to taste

3 cups cooked rice

½ cup chopped parsley, for garnish

½ cup steamed snow peas, for garnish

8 sections lemon

1. Spray a large nonstick saucepan with extra-virgin olive oil. Sauté the onions, garlic, and celery on medium-high heat for about 5 minutes, until the onions soften. Add the saffron, thyme, red pepper, and asparagus. Cover and sauté on medium heat, stirring frequently, for 5 minutes.

2. Add the peas, zucchini, tomatoes, and seitan. Stir well, cover, and simmer for 6 to 8 minutes, or until the vegetables are tender. Add sea salt and freshly milled black pepper to taste.

3. To serve the paella, first put the rice in individual bowls. Top with the vegetables and their juices. Sprinkle with chopped parsley and steamed snow peas. Squeeze fresh lemon juice over the top.

Amount Per Serving

Calories 352   Calories from Fat 27   Total Calories From: Fat 8% Protein 10% Carb. 82%

Vitamin A 36%   Vitamin C 111%   Iron 27%

Spinach Noodles Italiano

The longer you cook the sauce for this dish, the sweeter the onion and garlic become!

6 SERVINGS

extra-virgin olive oil cooking spray

1 onion, chopped

4 cloves garlic, minced

2 tablespoons fresh oregano, chopped

2 tablespoons fresh basil, chopped

1 tablespoon fresh thyme, chopped

6 to 8 tomatoes, chopped

1 cup tomato purée

1 pound whole-wheat spinach noodles

1. Brown onion and garlic in a nonstick saucepan that has been lightly coated with olive oil cooking spray. As onion begins to brown, stir in a little water to moisten and continue browning.

2. When onions are soft, stir in herbs, chopped tomatoes, and tomato purée. Simmer sauce uncovered for 1 hour or longer if possible.

3. Ten minutes before serving, cook noodles until tender, drain, and rinse. Serve with sauce.

Amount Per Serving

Calories 354   Calories from Fat 34   Total Calories From: Fat 9% Protein 15% Carb. 76%

Vitamin A 28%   Vitamin C 82%   Iron 26%

Penne Royal Supreme

In this version of a classic pasta dish from Northern Italy, veggie ground round takes the place of the usual ground beef, and tubular penne stands in for the traditional spaghetti. The result is a chunky, "meaty" red sauce that clings deliciously to the hollow pasta and is even more satisfying than the original. Serve with a green salad and Italian bread.

6 SERVINGS

1 onion, diced

2 12-ounce packages veggie ground round or tempeh

3 cloves garlic, minced

½ cup nonalcoholic red wine*

10 plum tomatoes, coarsely chopped

1 tablespoon brown sugar

¼ cup Italian parsley, chopped

1 pound eggless penne pasta, or substitute other pasta of choice

soy parmesan cheese, optional garnish

1. Spray a large nonstick saucepan with extra-virgin olive oil cooking spray and heat over medium-high heat.

Add onion and veggie ground round. Sauté until browned, about 8 minutes. Add a little water as needed to prevent burning. Add the garlic and sauté for an additional 30 seconds.

2. Stir in the wine, tomatoes, brown sugar, and parsley. Lower the heat and simmer for 30 minutes.

3. Meanwhile, cook the pasta until al dente. Drain.

4. Toss pasta with sauce. Top with soy parmesan, if desired.

*Nonalcoholic wine can be purchased in the wine section of supermarkets, or at your local wine store.

Amount Per Serving

Calories 302   Calories from Fat 43   Total Calories From: Fat 14% Protein 13% Carb. 73%

Vitamin A 17%   Vitamin C 39%   Iron 22%

Pasta with Fresh Tomatoes, Basil, and Roasted Garlic

I like to make this delicately spiced dish in the summer when fresh, ripe tomatoes are sweet and plentiful. The addition of fresh basil and roasted garlic adds a gourmet touch.

4 SERVINGS

10 cloves garlic

2 cups plum tomatoes, diced

⅓ cup fresh basil, chopped

1 teaspoon capers

1 tablespoon extra-virgin olive oil

1 tablespoon balsamic vinegar

½ pound whole wheat pasta of your choice

1. Place unpeeled garlic cloves in a small baking dish and roast at 350° F until soft and lightly colored, 15 to 20 minutes. Remove each clove as it is done. When cool enough to handle, peel and smash gently with the flat side of a knife.

2. Place tomatoes in a quart saucepan. Add roasted garlic and cook for 5-6 minutes. Remove from heat and add basil, capers, oil, and vinegar. Let stand at least 20 minutes to allow flavors to blend.

3. Bring a large pot of water to a boil. Cook pasta until al dente. Drain well and add to tomato mixture. Toss to mix and coat. Serve warm or at room temperature.

Amount Per Serving

Calories 36   Calories from Fat 3   Total Calories From: Fat 9% Protein 14% Carb. 77%

Vitamin A 12%   Vitamin C 330%   Iron 4%

Buffy's Rice-Lentils Medley

Onions, coriander, garlic, and cumin lend this otherwise earthy rice-lentil dish an exotic flavor. You might want to make the rice and lentils ahead, and do the topping just 10 minutes before serving for a quick and simple meal.

6 SERVINGS

1½ cups brown rice, uncooked

1½ cups dried lentils

1 bay leaf

6 cups water or Basic Vegetable Stock (see page 78)

1 teaspoon extra-virgin olive oil

3 onions, sliced into thin rounds

¾ teaspoon sea salt or salt substitute

4 cloves garlic, minced

1½ teaspoons coriander

¾ teaspoon cumin

¼ teaspoon cayenne pepper

1. Clean, rinse, and drain rice and lentils. Place in a 4-quart pot with bay leaf and water. Bring to a boil. Lower heat and simmer 45 minutes.

2. Just 10 minutes before serving, heat a nonstick skillet or wok. Add the oil, onions, and a pinch of salt and sauté.

3. When onions soften and begin to brown, add the garlic and spices and remaining sea salt. Cover and cook until onions are golden and have begun to caramelize.

4. When rice and lentils are finished, remove from heat and take out the bay leaf. Serve rice and lentils topped with the onion mixture.

Amount Per Serving

Calories 401   Calories from Fat 27   Total Calories From: Fat 7% Protein 19% Carb. 74%

Vitamin A 2%   Vitamin C 21%   Iron 32%

Larry's Lentil Loaf

This wonderful meatless loaf not only makes a delicious hot dinner, but the leftovers are great stuffed in Homemade Tortillas (see page 212) for quick burritos.

8 SERVINGS

1 crusty loaf of whole-grain bread
(9-inch round)

2 cups apple cider

1 cup dried lentils

2 carrots, finely chopped

1 bay leaf

2 stalks celery, finely chopped

1 large onion, finely chopped

1 sweet green pepper,
finely chopped

2 cloves garlic, minced

1 tablespoon extra-virgin olive oil

½ cup low-fat soy cheddar cheese

½ cup fresh parsley, minced

¼ cup egg substitute

1 teaspoon dried thyme

1. Using a serrated knife, horizontally cut the top quarter from the bread. Wrap the top in foil and set aside.

2. Scoop out the soft interior of the bread, leaving a ¾-inch to 1-inch shell. Do not puncture the sides or bottom of the loaf. Reserve the removed crumbs for another use. Set aside the hollow loaf.

3. In a 3-quart saucepan, combine the cider, lentils, carrots, and bay leaf. Bring to a boil. Reduce heat and simmer, partially covered, for 35 to 40 minutes, or until the lentils are tender and all the liquid has been absorbed. Stir occasionally to prevent sticking. Discard the bay leaf.

4. In a large nonstick skillet, sauté the celery, onion, peppers, and garlic in the oil until softened, about 5 minutes. Add to the lentil mixture. Stir in the cheese, parsley, egg substitute, and thyme.

5. Spoon the lentils into the hollow loaf. Wrap the loaf in foil and place on a baking sheet. Bake at 350° F for 1 hour. Add the foil-wrapped top to the oven and bake another 5 minutes.

continued overleaf

6. Unwrap the filled loaf and place it on a large serving platter. Unwrap the top and put it in place. To serve, scoop out the lentil mixture. Then cut the bread with a serrated knife and serve with the lentils.

Amount Per Serving

Calories 235   Calories from Fat 45   Total Calories From: Fat 19% Protein 19% Carb. 62%

Vitamin A 115%   Vitamin C 56%   Iron 22%

Tuscan Beans

This is great served with steamed spinach on the side.

4 SERVINGS

extra-virgin olive oil cooking spray

8 cloves garlic, finely minced

2 tablespoons fresh sage, finely chopped

1 teaspoon fresh thyme

2 cups fresh tomatoes

1½ tablespoons fresh lemon juice

2½ cups cooked white beans (Great Northern) or 2 15-ounce cans

sea salt or salt substitute, to taste

freshly milled black pepper, to taste

1. Lightly coat a nonstick saucepan with extra-virgin olive oil spray. Combine the garlic, sage, and thyme and sauté on medium-low heat for several minutes.

2. Add the tomatoes, lemon juice, and beans and continue to cook for 5–10 minutes longer. Add salt and pepper to taste.

Amount Per Serving

Calories 162   Calories from Fat 8   Total Calories From: Fat 5% Protein 23% Carb. 72%

Vitamin A 13%   Vitamin C 30%   Iron 19%

Taxco Black Beans and Rice Supreme

This delicious dish can literally be made in minutes.

4 SERVINGS

1 teaspoon extra-virgin olive oil

2 sweet red peppers, finely chopped

1 large onion, finely chopped

2 cloves garlic, minced

¼ teaspoon dried thyme

2 cups cooked black beans

2 tablespoons apple cider vinegar

2 cups hot cooked rice of choice
(see page 71)

soy sour cream (optional)

Red Chili Paste
(optional; see page 196)

1. Heat the oil in a large nonstick skillet or wok. Add the peppers, onions, celery, garlic, and thyme. Sauté over medium heat until the vegetables are tender, about 10 minutes.

2. Add the beans and vinegar. Cook until the beans are hot, about 3 minutes.

3. To serve, divide the rice among shallow bowls. Top with beans and soy sour cream if desired, or spice it up with Red Chili Paste.

Amount Per Serving

Calories 569   Calories from Fat 47   Total Calories From: Fat 8% Protein 13% Carb. 79%

Vitamin A 42%   Vitamin C 127%   Iron 37%

Spicy Veggie Chili Beans

If you plan ahead to cook the beans, the rest of this recipe is a snap and it has the added bonus of being almost fat-free. For those times when there is simply no time to plan ahead, use a good brand of well-rinsed canned beans and sauté the garlic and onions before combining and simmering all of the ingredients. Serve with Basque Spanish Rice (see page 181) and a green salad.

4 SERVINGS

1½ cups kidney beans, uncooked

extra-virgin olive oil cooking spray

1½ cups onion, chopped

2 cloves garlic, minced

½ green bell pepper, chopped

½ teaspoon onion powder

½ teaspoon garlic powder

1½ teaspoons cumin

½ teaspoon oregano

1½ teaspoons chili powder

1¾ cups hot water

1 cup tomato purée

1 tablespoon cider vinegar

2 green onions, chopped, for garnish

1. Soak dried beans, covered with water, overnight. Drain, then rinse.

2. Bring beans to a boil. Cover and cook very slowly, stirring occasionally so beans do not stick and burn. Cook until beans are tender, approximately 2 ½ hours.

3. While beans are cooking, spray a nonstick skillet or wok with extra-virgin olive oil cooking spray and sauté the onion, garlic, and bell pepper, adding a little water, if needed, to prevent burning. Stir in spices and seasonings, and continue cooking until onions and bell pepper are softened and moisture is absorbed. This should take 5 to 7 minutes.

4. Stir hot water, tomato purée, and sautéed vegetables into pot with cooked beans and continue to cook for 5 minutes.

5. Ten minutes before serving, add vinegar. Serve garnished with green onions on top of each serving.

Amount Per Serving

Calories 303   Calories from Fat 6   Total Calories From: Fat 2% Protein 25% Carb. 73%

Vitamin A 23%   Vitamin C 63%   Iron 44%

Spicy Refried Beans

Inspired by refried beans we had in a local restaurant, this dish is easy to make and satisfying to eat. It's also great stuffed in a fat-free tortilla shell.

6 SERVINGS

1 cup pinto beans

3 cups water, or more as needed to keep beans from burning

½ medium onion, chopped

½ cup sweet red bell pepper, diced

1 bay leaf

2 cloves garlic, minced

1 teaspoon chili powder

½ teaspoon cumin

½ teaspoon oregano

½ teaspoon thyme

½ cup tomato purée

1 teaspoon red wine vinegar

sea salt or salt substitute, to taste

1. Soak the pinto beans in water to cover by 2 inches, at least 8 hours or overnight.

2. Drain and rinse presoaked beans. Put beans in a pot and add the water and bay leaf. Bring beans to a boil, cover, then reduce heat and simmer slowly until tender, approximately 2½ hours.

3. Meanwhile, sauté onion and bell pepper in a large nonstick frying pan. After 5 minutes add the garlic and continue to sauté until onions are soft. Add water as needed to prevent onions and garlic from burning. Add the chili powder, cumin, oregano, thyme, tomato purée, and red wine vinegar.
Set aside.

4. When beans are cooked, add the seasoned onion and garlic mixture. Simmer for a few minutes before serving.

Amount Per Serving

Calories 47   Calories from Fat 3   Total Calories From: Fat 6% Protein 18% Carb. 76%

Vitamin A 8%   Vitamin C 15%   Iron 6%

Red Kidney Beans with Rice

This makes a quick and easy delicious meal. Top with salsa. The leftovers can be heated and stuffed into pita bread for a tasty hot lunch.

6 SERVINGS

extra-virgin olive oil cooking spray

2 cups onions, chopped

2 tablespoons garlic, finely minced

1 cup carrots, diced

1 cup celery, diced

1 cup red or green bell peppers, diced

1 teaspoon dried marjoram

1 teaspoon dried basil

1 teaspoon dried oregano

½ teaspoon dried thyme

⅛ teaspoon cayenne pepper

3 cups fresh or canned tomatoes, diced

1½ cups cooked or canned kidney beans

1 tablespoon Dijon mustard

1 tablespoon brown sugar

sea salt or salt substitute, to taste

freshly milled black pepper, to taste

red onion, diced, or fresh parsley

3 cups cooked rice

1. Over medium heat, sauté onion and garlic in a nonstick soup pot coated with olive oil cooking spray until the onions are translucent. Add the carrots, celery, bell peppers, marjoram, basil, oregano, thyme, and cayenne. Cover and cook for another 5 to 10 minutes, stirring and adding water as needed to prevent burning.

2. When the vegetables are just tender, stir in the remaining ingredients. Simmer gently for 10 minutes. Adjust seasoning to taste. Serve over a half cup of rice in bowls as you would a stew and sprinkle red onion or parsley on top.

Amount Per Serving

Calories 227   Calories from Fat 7   Total Calories From: Fat 3% Protein 24% Carb. 73%

Vitamin A 115%   Vitamin C 54%   Iron 30%

Puerto Rican Rice and Beans

The savory blend of garlic, onions, and peppers with rice and beans makes this dish a delicious event. Add a tossed salad and a green vegetable and you have a meal fit for royalty.

6 SERVINGS

4 cups water

1 cup dried pinto beans

1 cup brown rice, uncooked

extra-virgin olive oil spray

½ onion, peeled and diced

2 cloves garlic, peeled, smashed, and chopped

1 sweet red pepper, cored, seeded, and diced

2 jalapeño peppers, seeded and diced

1 tablespoon fresh oregano, chopped

1 15-ounce can peeled plum tomatoes, drained with juice reserved

½ teaspoon sea salt or salt substitute

½ teaspoon freshly milled black pepper

3 tablespoons fresh cilantro, chopped

2 tablespoons capers

1. Place the water and pinto beans in a pressure cooker and cook for 20 minutes. Add the rice, and when the pressure cooker "hisses," cook for another 5 minutes.

2. While the rice and beans cook, sauté the onion and garlic until the onion becomes translucent. Add a bit of water to prevent burning if needed. Add the peppers, oregano, and tomatoes, stirring and chopping as you go. Add ¼ cup of the reserved tomato juice, half of the salt, and half of the pepper. Lower the heat and simmer 15 minutes.

3. After the rice and beans have cooked, stir in 2 tablespoons of the cilantro, the capers, and the remaining salt and pepper. Serve garnished with the remaining cilantro.

Amount Per Serving

Calories 48   Calories from Fat 3   Total Calories From: Fat 6% Protein 18% Carb. 76%

Vitamin A 47%   Vitamin C 103%   Iron 6%

Down Home Baked Beans

This is a staple for summer picnics. The beans take a while to prepare, but the flavor is worth it. Just plan ahead for this dish.

8 SERVINGS

1 cup dry navy beans

extra-virgin olive oil cooking spray

1 large onion, diced

2 cloves garlic, finely minced

2 cups water

¼ cup dry sherry

1 bay leaf

3 tablespoons molasses

2 tablespoons brown sugar

½ teaspoon dry mustard

⅛ teaspoon ground cinnamon

⅛ teaspoon ground nutmeg

⅛ teaspoon ground ginger

1 tablespoon lemon juice

1 8-ounce can salt-free tomato sauce

1. Soak the navy beans in water to cover by 2 inches, at least 8 hours or overnight.

2. Heat saucepan over medium heat and spray with extra-virgin olive oil cooking spray. Add the onion and garlic and cook about 5 minutes, until the onions are softened. Remove from heat.

3. Rinse and drain the beans. Put the beans in a large oven-proof pot. Add all ingredients except the tomato sauce. Mix well, cover, and place in the refrigerator for 12–24 hours.

4. To bake, preheat oven to 350° F. Add the tomato sauce to the beans, and place the pot of beans in the preheated oven. Bake 4 hours, covered. Check beans after 3 hours and, if necessary, add a little more water so that beans are covered with liquid.

5. Remove and discard bay leaf before serving. Serve hot or at room temperature.

Amount Per Serving

Calories 176   Calories from Fat 16   Total Calories From: Fat 9% Protein 11% Carb. 80%

Vitamin A 10%   Vitamin C 26%   Iron 19%

Tofu with Spicy Vegetables

This colorful medley of vegetables and tofu is as tasty as it looks. If you're lucky enough to have any left over, it's also great stuffed into pita bread for a quick and easy delicious sandwich.

4 SERVINGS

1 onion, thinly sliced

1 sweet red pepper,
cut into 2-inch strips

2 stalks celery,
thinly sliced diagonally

4 cloves garlic, minced

1 tablespoon ginger root,
peeled and minced

1 tablespoon chili pepper, minced

1 tablespoon extra-virgin olive oil

½ cup mushrooms, thinly sliced

¾ cup broccoli florets

¾ cup cauliflower florets

¼ cup peas

1 cup low-fat tofu, cubed

¼ cup cooking sherry

1 tablespoon tamari soy sauce

1 tablespoon sugar

1 tablespoon cornstarch
blended with 2 tablespoons water

2 cups brown rice, cooked

1. Heat a large nonstick skillet or wok over medium heat. Sauté the onion, red pepper, celery, garlic, ginger, and chili pepper in the oil for 5 minutes. Add the mushrooms, broccoli, cauliflower, peas, and tofu. Stir to combine.

2. Add the cooking sherry, soy sauce, and sugar. Cover and cook for 3 to 4 minutes, or until the vegetables are crisp-tender. Add the cornstarch mixture and stir until thickened. Remove from heat and put on warmed serving platter.

3. Serve over hot brown rice.

Amount Per Serving

Calories 519   Calories from Fat 49   Total Calories From: Fat 9% Protein 10% Carb. 81%

Vitamin A 45%   Vitamin C 182%   Iron 39%

Scrambled Tofu Jalapeño

This colorful dish makes a hearty Sunday breakfast. For variety, use vegetables other than those called for in the recipe. Serve with a fresh fruit salad for brunch.

4 SERVINGS

8 ounces low-fat tofu, drained

1 jalapeño pepper, chopped

1 red bell pepper, chopped

1 green bell pepper, chopped

2 tablespoons parsley, chopped

2 green onion, including tops, chopped

2 tomatoes, diced

1 teaspoon onion powder

1 teaspoon nutritional yeast (see glossary)

¼ teaspoon turmeric

freshly milled black pepper, to taste

4 whole wheat tortillas (optional)

4 tablespoons salsa (optional)

1. Mash the drained tofu with a fork into the consistency of scrambled eggs and place it in a nonstick skillet over medium heat. Stir in the remaining ingredients and cover.

2. Slowly simmer all ingredients for 8–10 minutes. Then simmer uncovered for 10 additional minutes. Serve immediately. Serve wrapped in whole wheat tortillas topped with salsa, if desired.

Amount Per Serving

Calories 179   Calories from Fat 29   Total Calories From: Fat 16% Protein 22% Carb. 62%

Vitamin A 36%   Vitamin C 94%   Iron 40%

Rice Tofu Stir-Fry

When I have leftover rice, this is one of the first dishes I think of making. It's always a hit with family and friends, plus it's quick and easy to prepare.

2 SERVINGS

10 ½ ounces firm low-fat tofu, drained and cubed

¼ cup tamari soy sauce

¼ cup rice wine vinegar

1 teaspoon sesame oil

1 cup carrots, shredded

½ cup green onion, sliced

¼ cup fresh ginger root, sliced

1 cup brown rice, cooked

1. Combine the tofu, soy sauce, vinegar, and sesame oil. Marinate in the refrigerator a minimum of 1 hour.

2. Heat all the marinated ingredients in a wok. Add the carrots, scallions, and ginger. Stir-fry until vegetables are tender but still crisp.

3. Add the rice and stir-fry to heat through. Serve.

Amount Per Serving

Calories 481   Calories from Fat 72   Total Calories From: Fat 15% Protein 9% Carb. 76%

Vitamin A 312%   Vitamin C 16%   Iron 22%

No-Beef Stroganoff

This version of a classic is quick to make and very delicious. Serve over whole wheat cous-cous, noodles, quinoa, or brown rice with a hot vegetable and green salad on the side.

4 SERVINGS

extra-virgin olive oil cooking spray

¼ cup mirin (see glossary)

4 tablespoons tamari soy sauce

1¼ cups soymilk

1½ cups sweet onion, finely diced

3 cloves garlic, finely minced

1 teaspoon fresh thyme

1 teaspoon fresh oregano

1 large carrot,
cut into 2-inch matchsticks

1 sweet red pepper,
cut into 2-inch matchsticks

1 8-ounce package tempeh,
cut into ¼-inch strips

3 tablespoons whole wheat pastry flour

freshly milled black pepper, to taste

pasta or grain of choice

1. Mix mirin, soy sauce, and soymilk together and set aside.

2. Lightly coat a large nonstick skillet with extra-virgin olive oil cooking spray. Add onion, garlic, thyme, and oregano. Sauté until onion is soft. Add carrots, pepper, and tempeh and cook until the tempeh starts to become golden, stirring constantly to prevent burning.

3. Add the flour, stirring it in to coat the vegetables thoroughly.

4. Slowly add the mirin mixture, stirring as you go to make a nice gravy. Season to taste with the freshly milled black pepper.

5. Put mixture into a casserole dish and bake for 30 minutes. Serve over rice, quinoa, noodles, or couscous.

Amount Per Serving

Calories 226	Calories from Fat 55	Total Calories From: Fat 24% Protein 29% Carb. 47%
		Vitamin A 156% Vitamin C 71% Iron 13%

Mad Dog Tempeh Loaf

Tempeh, a traditional Indonesian food made from cultured whole soybeans that are pressed into thin cakes, can be found in the frozen foods section of most natural food stores and many local supermarkets. This hearty loaf makes great sandwich fillings, or serve the loaf buffet-style with crackers or crudités.

8 SERVINGS

extra-virgin olive oil cooking spray

16 ounces tempeh

½ cup onion, finely diced

2 cloves garlic, minced

½ cup celery, diced

1 tablespoon nutritional yeast
(see glossary)

2 tablespoons wheat germ

½ cup egg substitute

1 cup dry bread crumbs, or ½ cup bread crumbs and ½ cup raw rolled oats

1 tablespoon Worcestershire sauce

⅓ cup catsup

½ teaspoon dried oregano

½ teaspoon dried marjoram

½ teaspoon dried thyme

½ teaspoon dried basil

1 teaspoon sea salt or salt substitute

½ teaspoon freshly milled black pepper

4 ounces tofu cheddar cheese (optional)

1. Mix all ingredients. If mixture seems too dry, add a little water as needed.

2. Spray a glass or nonstick metal baking pan with olive oil spray and press loaf into pan. If using cheese, cut into several small sticks. Insert sticks straight down into loaf at several intervals. As baking proceeds, these melt internally and across the top. Bake in preheated 350° F oven for approximately 45 minutes, or until fully cooked and browned. Remove from oven.

3. Cool for 10 minutes before slicing. Serve with potatoes, steamed green beans or carrots, and a crisp raw vegetable salad.

Amount Per Serving

Calories 195   Calories from Fat 47   Total Calories From: Fat 24% Protein 27% Carb. 49%

Vitamin A 10%   Vitamin C 5%   Iron 12%

Hungarian Goulash

My husband gave me the idea for this delicious vegetarian version of the old standard. You'll never miss the meat. Serve over eggless noodles with a steamed green vegetable and a salad, and your meal is complete.

6 SERVINGS

1 tablespoon extra-virgin olive oil

1 onion, diced

2 12-ounce packages veggie ground round (I like Yves brand) or use tempeh

6 cloves garlic, minced

2 tablespoons paprika

3 cups Basic Vegetable Stock (see page 78) or water with vegetable bouillon added

½ cup nonalcoholic dry white wine*

2 cups strained sauerkraut

8 button mushrooms, quartered

3 tablespoons caraway seeds

12 ounces flat eggless noodles

1 cup soy sour cream (optional)

1. Heat the oil in a large nonstick saucepan over high heat and sauté the onion for about 7 minutes. Stir frequently to prevent the onion from burning. Add the veggie ground round and stir for 4 minutes, making sure it is well blended with the onion.

2. Add the garlic and paprika, stirring until the onion is well coated with paprika, about 1 minute.

3. Add the stock, wine, sauerkraut, mushrooms, and caraway seeds. Reduce the heat and simmer for 30 minutes.

4. While the goulash is simmering, cook the noodles. Set aside and keep warm.

5. If you are using the sour cream, add it to the goulash by spoonfuls, stirring after each addition, and simmer for 5 minutes. Do not bring it to a boil.

6. Spoon the goulash over the hot noodles and serve immediately.

*Nonalcoholic wine can be found in the beverage or wine section of most good supermarkets or wine stores today.

Amount Per Serving

Calories 337   Calories from Fat 63   Total Calories From: Fat 18% Protein 14% Carb. 68%

Vitamin A 32%   Vitamin C 28%   Iron 31%

Buffy's Egg Fu-Yung

This one-dish meal is a favorite of my husband and the Asian students we frequently host. It's a great way to use leftover rice.

4 SERVINGS

extra-virgin olive oil cooking spray

1 egg white

¾ cup egg substitute

8 button mushrooms, sliced, or 2 Chinese dried mushrooms, washed and soaked for 25 minutes

6 green onions, including tops, sliced diagonally

½ cup sweet green pepper, diced

⅓ cup bamboo shoots, thinly sliced

½ cup snow peas, sliced diagonally

2 cups bean sprouts

1 cup brown rice, cooked

2 tablespoons tamari soy sauce

2 tablespoons dry sherry

1 teaspoon sesame oil

sea salt or salt substitute, to taste

freshly ground black pepper, to taste

1. Combine the beaten egg white and egg substitute and mix with a little salt. Heat a non-stick skillet and spray it with extra-virgin olive oil. Add the beaten egg mixture and stir until just set. Remove and set aside.

2. Heat nonstick wok or skillet. Add mushrooms, scallions, and green bell pepper. Stir-fry for 2 minutes. Add the bamboo shoots, snow peas, and bean sprouts. Stir-fry for 1 minute.

3. Add the rice and remaining ingredients. Mix well, heating the rice thoroughly. Season to taste with salt and pepper. Stir in the eggs and serve.

Amount Per Serving

Calories 211   Calories from Fat 14   Total Calories From: Fat 6% Protein 12% Carb. 82%

Vitamin A 2%   Vitamin C 34%   Iron 17%

Potato-Tomato Casserole

We first tasted this wonderfully simple country-style dish when visiting Tuscany in the fall of 1995. We've loved it ever since.

4 SERVINGS

4 pounds thin-skinned potatoes, unpeeled

4 tomatoes, coarsely chopped

1 onion, thinly sliced

4 cloves garlic, finely chopped

2 tablespoons fresh thyme

1 bay leaf

½ cup Basic Vegetable Stock, (see page 78)

sea salt or salt substitute, to taste

freshly milled black pepper, to taste

1. Preheat oven to 375° F.

2. Wash potatoes and cut into 1-inch cubes.
Put vegetable stock into a deep baking dish. Add the potatoes, tomatoes, onion, garlic, herbs, sea salt, and pepper and stir gently to mix.

3. Put vegetable mixture on top rack of preheated oven and bake for about 1 hour or until the potatoes are tender and the stock has been absorbed. Serve hot, directly from the dish.

Amount Per Serving

Calories 551   Calories from Fat 11   Total Calories From: Fat 2% Protein 9% Carb. 89%

Vitamin A 17%   Vitamin C 175%   Iron 38%

Stuffed Acorn Squash

This is a favorite wintertime dish at our home. I grow my own acorn squash, and they can be stored in a cool place throughout the winter.

4 SERVINGS

2 acorn squash, cut in half and seeded

1 cup brown rice, cooked

¼ cup raisins

1 Granny Smith apple, chopped

½ cup soft whole-grain bread crumbs

¼ cup onion, finely chopped

⅛ teaspoon cayenne pepper

2 teaspoons curry powder

1 teaspoon coriander

2 tablespoons apple juice concentrate, plus 4 teaspoons to sprinkle on each half acorn squash before baking

4 sprigs of fresh coriander, for garnish

1. Preheat oven to 350° F.

2. Place halves of acorn squash, cavity facing down, in a baking pan with ½ inch of water. Bake for 30 minutes or until squash is tender when center is pierced with a fork.

3. While squash is baking, mix together the next 9 ingredients. Spoon mixture into baked squash halves. Pour 1 teaspoon apple juice concentrate over each, sprinkle with coriander, and bake 30 minutes or until hot and light brown on top. Remove from oven and serve.

Amount Per Serving

Calories 405   Calories from Fat 23   Total Calories From: Fat 5% Protein 8% Carb. 87%

Vitamin A 17%   Vitamin C 58%   Iron 20%

Side Dishes

▼

Side dishes add the finishing touches to well-planned meals. They supplement and complement main dishes, offering appealing contrasts in appearance and texture. Some recipes are even hearty enough to stand on their own as light meals. Those that feature whole-grain pasta or rice are high in carbohydrates and fiber, helping you to feel pleasantly satisfied when the meal ends. Most also include vegetables, providing essential nutrients. For variety, try preparing and serving a side dish such as Vegetarian Stir-Fry or Over-Stuffed Baked Potato for a luxurious lunch. For the most part, you can eat as many servings of vegetables as you like each day. Be sure to include plenty of cruciferous vegetables as well as tomatoes to give your body a strong daily dose of the cancer-fighting substances found in these foods.

Keep Nutrients in Cooked Vegetables

It isn't boiling that drains nutrients from vegetables — it's preboiling. When water temperature is between 60° F and 90° F, certain enzymes go to work that cause vegetables to deteriorate. The best solution is to eat vegetables raw, or steam them, whenever possible. But if you're going to boil them, bring the water to a full boil first and then add the vegetables. The higher temperature neutralizes the enzymes, reducing deterioration and nutrient loss.

Steamy Steamed Vegetables

Steamed vegetables are delicious, and quick and easy to make. Plus, steaming is one of the best ways of preserving the nutrients in vegetables. One of my favorite steamed vegetable combinations is corn on the cob, a wedge of cabbage, and broccoli or cauliflower florets. Just add salt and pepper to taste, or your favorite fat-free dressing or sauce.

Steaming consists simply of cooking food in a tightly covered pot over, but not immersed in, a small amount of boiling water. The steam cooks the food. Some simple guidelines to follow when steaming are:

- *Keep the cooking time short. You can do this by cutting dense vegetables into thin pieces.*
- *Check for doneness by piercing with the tip of a sharp knife.*
- *When vegetables are ready, immediately uncover the pot and remove from heat, to stop the cooking process.*
- *Since every vegetable requires a different steaming time, it is best to steam them separately, or add faster-steaming vegetables after slower ones have partially cooked.*
- *Make sure the pot you use has a tight-fitting lid.*

1. Trim and cut vegetables as required.

2. Preheat the steamer. You may use a pot specifically designed for steaming, or improvise by placing a steaming basket in the bottom of one of your general-purpose pots. Add about ½ inch of water to the pot.

3. Place the steaming basket with the vegetables in the pot, cover, and bring to a boil over high heat.

4. When steam begins to escape, reduce heat to low and start timing. Root vegetables such as carrots, potatoes, and turnips may take up to 15 minutes or more, depending on how thickly they are sliced, while greens such as mustard or collard take about 5 minutes; broccoli and cauliflower, 6 to 7 minutes.

5. Remove vegetables from the steamer as soon as they reach the desired tenderness.

6. Dress the steamed vegetables with your choice of nonfat sauce or dressing just before serving.

Below is a colorful array of lightly steamed vegetables which could serve an interesting side dish or a hearty main dish for two.

2 carrots, cut into ¼-inch rounds

2 cups cauliflower florets

10 string beans, trimmed

2 yellow squash, cut into ¼-inch rounds

2 zucchini, cut into ¼-inch rounds

2 cups broccoli florets

1. Bring water to a boil over high heat in a steamer. Fit the basket into the steamer and put in the carrots, cauliflower, and string beans. Cover and cook for 3 minutes. Add the yellow squash, zucchini, and broccoli. Re-cover and cook for 2 minutes more.

2. Transfer the vegetables to a warm platter and serve dressed with your choice of nonfat sauce or dressing.

Amount Per Serving

Calories 156	Calories from Fat 11	Total Calories From: Fat 7% Protein 22% Carb. 71%
		Vitamin A 454% Vitamin C 312% Iron 17%

Roasted Root Vegetables

Medium-size vegetables are best for this dish since they have the maturity needed for flavor, yet are small enough to be tender. Choose your favorites, such as sweet potatoes, small onions or whole shallots, carrots, turnips, parsnips, beets, or thin-skinned potatoes. Roasted vegetables can be served on rice, couscous, bulgur, beds of steamed greens, or treated as a side dish.

6 SERVINGS

2 ½ pounds mixed root vegetables

1 head garlic, unpeeled and separated into cloves

3 bay leaves

1 tablespoon fresh thyme

6 short rosemary sprigs or 10 sage leaves

sea salt or salt substitute, to taste

freshly milled black pepper, to taste

extra-virgin olive oil cooking spray

1. Preheat the oven to 400° F. Peel the vegetables, onions, or shallots. Cut everything into pieces roughly the same size except for turnips, parsnips, and sweet potatoes, which cook faster and can be slightly larger than the rest. Toss the vegetables, garlic, and herbs to coat lightly, then season with salt and pepper.

2. Spray a nonstick baking sheet with olive oil cooking spray.

Put everything in one layer on a baking sheet. Add 3 to 5 tablespoons of water to the bottom of the pan. Bake, uncovered, in the top third of the oven for 40 to 60 minutes, turning the vegetables as needed. Remove from oven.

3. Serve hot with your favorite nonfat sauce or balsamic vinegar sprinkled over the vegetables as soon as they come out of the oven.

For variety, replace the herbs with either Jamaican Marinade or Caribbean Marinade (see pages 199 and 201). Also, this is a great time to roast extra garlic or onions for use in other dishes.

Amount Per Serving

Calories 128   Calories from Fat 3   Total Calories From: Fat 3% Protein 17% Carb. 80%

Vitamin A 163%   Vitamin C 11%   Iron 11%

Basic Oven-Roasted Vegetables

4 SERVINGS

4 small red potatoes,
(½ pound), scrubbed

4 carrots, peeled

4 zucchini

1 yellow bell pepper, cleaned
with stem and seeds removed

1 red bell pepper, cleaned
with stem and seeds removed

½ cup Basic Vegetable Stock
(see page 78) or water

1 tablespoon coarse sea salt
or salt substitute

freshly milled black pepper,
to taste

1. Preheat oven to 400° F. Cut potatoes into 1½-inch rounds. Cut carrots, zucchini, and peppers into 1-inch chunks.

2. Arrange potatoes and carrots on a baking sheet and drizzle with ⅓ cup broth. Season with salt and pepper. Roast for 20 minutes.

3. Add zucchini and bell peppers to baking sheet. Drizzle on the remaining broth and season with salt and pepper. Roast another 20 minutes or until all vegetables are browned and tender. Serve warm or at room temperature.

Amount Per Serving

Calories 124   Calories from Fat 6   Total Calories From: Fat 5% Protein 12% Carb. 83%

Vitamin A 438%   Vitamin C 105%   Iron 10%

Over-Stuffed Baked Potato

A dish we enjoyed when eating at a local restaurant inspired this recipe, but their version was loaded with cheese on top. Ours is much healthier, and just as good!

4 SERVINGS

extra-virgin olive oil cooking spray

4 baked potatoes, cooked
and cut in half lengthwise

1 bunch broccoli, cut into small florets

6 cloves garlic, finely minced

⅛ teaspoon red pepper flakes

¼ cup nonfat soymilk

sea salt and
freshly milled black pepper, to taste

6 black olives, cut in quarters
and added to the mashed potato
broccoli mixture (optional)

1. Steam the broccoli until crisp-tender.

2. Sauté the garlic and red pepper flakes in a nonstick pan lightly sprayed with extra virgin olive oil cooking spray, for 1 minute. Remove from heat.

3. Scoop out the potato pulp and mash it with the garlic, soymilk, salt, and pepper. Add the broccoli and black olives if desired, and stir it into the mashed potatoes. Refill the potato skins and bake for 30 minutes.

Amount Per Serving

Calories 48   Calories from Fat 4   Total Calories From: Fat 8% Protein 30% Carb. 62%

Vitamin A 35%   Vitamin C 179%   Iron 6%

Mashed Potatoes and Turnips with Garlic

This is a great variation on the classic mashed potatoes.

6 SERVINGS

extra-virgin olive oil cooking spray

1 onion, finely chopped

3 large heads garlic

1¼ pounds turnips,
peeled and quartered

1½ pounds large russet potatoes,
peeled and quartered

1¾ cups Basic Vegetable Stock
(see page 78)

¼ cup soymilk

sea salt or salt substitute, to taste

freshly milled white pepper, to taste

1. Spray a nonstick baking pan with olive oil cooking spray. Add onion. Cut unpeeled garlic heads into halves crosswise. Place, cut sides down, in pan with onion. Bake in 375° F oven for 40-45 minutes, stirring onions occasionally until they are browned and garlic is very tender when pierced in center. Set aside until garlic is cool enough to touch.

2. In a 4-quart pan, combine turnips, potatoes, and broth. Bring to a boil over high heat. Reduce heat, cover, and boil gently until vegetables are very tender when pierced and almost all broth has been absorbed (about 25 minutes).

3. Squeeze garlic from skins into a small bowl. Discard skins. Using the back of a spoon, mash garlic to a smooth paste. Mix in browned onions, then set mixture aside.

4. Transfer potato mixture to a large bowl. Using a potato masher, mash until smooth. Add milk and garlic-onion mixture. Whip until smooth and creamy. Season to taste with salt and white pepper, then transfer to a shallow 2-quart casserole. Broil about 4 inches below heat until top is golden brown, about 3 to 5 minutes.

You can bake the potatoes and turnips along with the onions to save a step and add a deeper flavor. The mashed potatoes take on a darker tint.

Amount Per Serving

Calories 167	Calories from Fat 4	Total Calories From: Fat 3% Protein 10% Carb. 87%
		Vitamin A 0% Vitamin C 65% Iron 10%

Greek-Style Onions

My father was an onion farmer, so I ate onions often as a child. There are many and varied ways of fixing onions, but this is one of our favorite combinations. A menu including fresh spinach or other hot greens and these onions will be special enough for unexpected company or for any festive family celebration.

6 SERVINGS

1 cup red wine, with or without alcohol

4 tablespoons red wine vinegar

3 tablespoons tomato paste

3 tablespoons light brown sugar

1 teaspoon extra-virgin olive oil

2 cups water

2 ¼ pounds pearl onions, peeled

4 tender celery stalks, thinly sliced

4 ounces seedless raisins

sea salt or salt substitute, to taste

freshly milled black pepper, to taste

3 tablespoons parsley, chopped

1 loaf whole wheat French bread, toasted

1. Put the wine, vinegar, tomato paste, sugar, olive oil, and water into a pan and stir over low heat to dissolve the sugar.

2. Add the onions, celery, and raisins. Season with salt and pepper. Bring to a boil over moderate heat, stirring occasionally.

3. Cover the pan and simmer gently for 35 minutes, or until the onions are tender. Taste the sauce and adjust the seasoning if necessary.

4. Stir in 2 tablespoons of the parsley. Garnish with the remainder. Serve hot, with plenty of crusty whole wheat bread.

Amount Per Serving

Calories 135   Calories from Fat 10   Total Calories From: Fat 9% Protein 9% Carb. 82%

Vitamin A 7%   Vitamin C 25%   Iron 9%

Vegetarian Stir-Fry

This is quick, easy, and delicious as a side dish. The variety of vegetables used in this dish gives it an attractive colorful appearance and an interesting blend of textures.

6 SERVINGS

extra-virgin olive oil cooking spray

4 cloves garlic, finely minced

¼ cup sweet onion

⅓ cup carrots

1 cup Napa cabbage

1 cup broccoli florets

½ cup cauliflower florets

½ cup sweet red bell pepper

⅓ cup snow peas

⅓ cup mushrooms

¼ cup bean sprouts

1 tablespoon tamari soy sauce

1 tablespoon brown rice vinegar

1 tablespoon mirin (see glossary)

1 tablespoon oyster sauce (optional)

2 cups brown rice, cooked

1. Cut the vegetables into matchsticks. Heat a nonstick wok or large skillet, spray it with the extra-virgin olive oil cooking spray, and stir-fry the garlic for 30 seconds.

2. Add all remaining ingredients. Stir-fry for 4 minutes or until the vegetables are crisp-tender.

3. Serve with brown rice on a warmed serving platter.

Amount Per Serving

Calories 38   Calories from Fat 2   Total Calories From: Fat 4% Protein 19% Carb. 77%

Vitamin A 49%   Vitamin C 76%   Iron 4%

Pepper Stir-Fry

This colorful array of peppers is great served hot. However, if you are lucky enough to have any left over, serve chilled on a bed of lettuce or stuffed into pita bread for a quick, easy snack.

4 SERVINGS

extra-virgin olive oil cooking spray

3 cloves garlic, finely minced

3 tablespoons cooking sherry

1 green bell pepper,
cut into one-inch pieces

1 red bell pepper,
cut into one-inch pieces

1 yellow bell pepper,
cut into one-inch pieces

¼ cup plus 2 tablespoons green onion, sliced

1½ teaspoons fresh basil, minced
(more if you want to use as garnish),
or ½ teaspoon dried whole basil

¼ teaspoon dill seeds

¼ teaspoon celery seeds

1. Heat a large nonstick skillet sprayed with extra-virgin olive oil cooking spray. Add the garlic and sauté for 30 seconds.

2. Add sherry, peppers, sliced green onions, basil, dill seeds, and celery seeds. Stir-fry 3 minutes or until vegetables are crisp-tender.

3. Transfer mixture to a warmed serving dish. Garnish with fresh basil, if desired.

Amount Per Serving

Calories 21   Calories from Fat 1   Total Calories From: Fat 6% Protein 13% Carb. 81%

Vitamin A 45%   Vitamin C 147%   Iron 3%

Stir-Fry Greens

Stir-fry greens are really simple and easy to make, and sooo delicious! You can stir-fry any one of these greens separately, or make up your own combinations. Either way, it'll be a hit!

4 SERVINGS

1 teaspoon mirin (see glossary)

1 teaspoon tamari soy sauce

1 teaspoon rice vinegar

1 teaspoon cornstarch, diluted with water

1 teaspoon oyster sauce (optional)

extra-virgin olive oil cooking spray

5 cloves garlic, minced

1 tablespoon ginger root, minced

2 tablespoons green onion, chopped

½ teaspoon red pepper flakes

10 cups bok choy, Napa cabbage, spinach, or other greens of choice, washed and sliced*

½ cup Stir-Fry Stock (see page 82)

1. Mix the mirin, soy sauce, and rice vinegar together (and oyster sauce, if using). Stir in the cornstarch mixture and set aside.

2. Heat a nonstick skillet or wok. Spray with extra-virgin olive oil cooking spray. Add garlic, ginger, green onion, and red pepper flakes. Stir-fry until the garlic is golden.
Remove from heat and set aside to sprinkle over the greens before serving.

3. Add the greens and stir-fry 1 to 2 minutes for young or delicate soft greens or 5 to 10 minutes for older or bulky greens. Add the stock.
Cover and steam about 2-3 minutes until greens are tender. Remove from heat.

4. Remove greens from wok and set them on a warmed platter. Add the soy sauce and cornstarch mixture to the juices left in the wok and heat until thickened. Pour thickened sauce over the greens. Sprinkle the reserved garlic, ginger, scallion, and red pepper flake mixture over the greens and serve immediately.

*Suggested greens: bok choy, mustard greens, romaine lettuce, Napa cabbage, spinach, and watercress

Amount Per Serving

Calories 50	Calories from Fat 6	Total Calories From: Fat 12% Protein 30% Carb. 58%
		Vitamin A 106% Vitamin C 136% Iron 10%

Sweet Kabocha Squash

A student whom we hosted from Japan introduced us to kabocha squash. It cooks very quickly, has a sweet mellow flavor, and is delicious!

4 SERVINGS

10 ounces kabocha squash,*
sweet mama squash,
or honey delight squash

1 cup Basic Vegetable Stock
(see page 78)

1 tablespoon brown sugar

1 tablespoon mirin (see glossary)

1 tablespoon low-sodium tamari soy sauce

1. Cut the squash into bite-size chunks, removing the skin around the corners and edges only.

2. Add the squash to the stock in a wide-bottomed saucepan and bring the mixture to a boil. Add the sugar and mirin. Make a cover out of parchment paper or aluminum foil and place over the mixture.

3. Cook until squash is tender. Add the soy sauce. When it returns to a boil, turn off heat and serve.

*Kabocha squash can be found in your Asian market.

Amount Per Serving

Calories 50   Calories from Fat 1   Total Calories From: Fat 3% Protein 10% Carb. 87%

Vitamin A 5%   Vitamin C 13%   Iron 3%

Snappy Spaghetti Squash

You can't miss this beautiful squash at the grocery store. It has a big, egg-shaped, yellow-skinned presence amongst the other vegetables. Make sure that its skin is hard, with no soft spots, decay, cracks, or bore holes. It should keep for about one month at room temperature.

4 SERVINGS

1 medium spaghetti squash

1 teaspoon extra-virgin olive oil

½ cup sweet green pepper, diced

½ cup sweet red pepper, diced

¼ cup onion, diced

¼ cup fresh coriander, minced

¼ cup Basic Vegetable Stock (see page 78)

1 teaspoon red wine vinegar

¼ teaspoon ground cumin

1 clove garlic, minced

1. Place the squash in a very large pot. Add water to cover. Bring to a boil and cook, uncovered, for 30 to 60 minutes, or until easily pierced with a fork. Drain, halve, and set aside until cool enough to handle. Discard the seeds. With a fork, separate the flesh into strands and place in a large bowl.

2. In a large nonstick skillet or wok, combine the oil, green pepper, red pepper, onion, coriander, stock, vinegar, cumin, and garlic. Cover and cook over medium heat for 5 minutes.

3. Add the squash and toss to combine. Cover and cook for 2 minutes to heat through and serve.

Spaghetti squash can also be cooked in a microwave:

▨ Select a small to medium spaghetti squash, about 1½ to 2 pounds, to serve four people.

▨ Cut the squash in half and remove the seeds.

▨ Place each half, cut side down, on a separate plate. The squash is moist enough to cook without any added liquid.

continued overleaf

■ Microwave each half separately on full power for 6 to 8 minutes, or until the flesh is tender and can be easily pulled from the shell in strands.

■ Remove the squash strands from the shell gently, using a fork.

For a variation on this dish, I like to make little pancake patties with the squash mixture and brown them on a nonstick grill.

Amount Per Serving

Calories 306   Calories from Fat 39   Total Calories From: Fat 13% Protein 6% Carb. 81%

Vitamin A 31%   Vitamin C 123%   Iron 21%

Marinated Raw Vegetables in Curry

This dish should be made ahead to allow the flavors to intensify. Serve this dish over your favorite grains or use couscous, which is not only delicious, but also quick and easy to prepare.

8 SERVINGS

2 tablespoons extra-virgin olive oil

¼ cup tamari soy sauce

1 teaspoon curry powder

¼ teaspoon ground cumin

3 tablespoons nutritional yeast*

2 cups water

1 onion, finely chopped

2 carrots, thinly sliced

1 cup cauliflower florets

1 cup broccoli, cut into small florets with stems peeled and sliced

1 red bell pepper, seeded and cut into thin strips

1 sweet green pepper, seeded and cut into thin strips

1 cup snow peas, diagonally sliced

1 cup butternut squash, peeled and cut into matchsticks

3 cups couscous, uncooked

4 cups boiling water

1. In a blender, combine the first 8 ingredients. Blend until mixture becomes a smooth sauce.

2. Mix together remaining vegetables in a large bowl. Pour in sauce, mixing with the vegetables making sure they all get coated, and allow vegetables to marinate for 3 hours or overnight.

3. Place couscous in a bowl and add boiling water. Cover and set aside for about 15 minutes, until water is absorbed.

4. Spoon marinated vegetables over couscous and serve.

*Nutritional yeast, available in health food stores, adds a rich, cheese-like flavor and creaminess to food. Do not confuse it with brewer's yeast, which has a characteristically bitter taste. Nutritional yeast is very high in protein and B vitamins. It can also be an effective thickening agent in dairy-free cream sauces and soups.

Amount Per Serving

Calories 339   Calories from Fat 37   Total Calories From: Fat 11% Protein 14% Carb. 75%

Vitamin A 144%   Vitamin C 105%   Iron 11%

Baked Oriental Eggplant

This recipe is an instant hit with everyone. It's hot and spicy and best served with mild dishes.

4 SERVINGS

1 pound eggplant, preferably Oriental*

Seasonings:

1 tablespoon ginger root, minced

2 cloves garlic, minced

¼ cup green onion, diced

Sauce:

2 tablespoons tamari soy sauce

2 tablespoons rice vinegar

¼ cup Basic Vegetable Stock (see page 78)

1 tablespoon Red Chili Paste (see page 196)

1 teaspoon honey

1. Cut the eggplant into ½-inch thick rounds. Place sliced eggplant onto a nonstick baking sheet and bake in a 350° F oven for 45 minutes.

2. Combine the seasonings in a small bowl and mix the ingredients for the sauce. While the eggplant is baking, place a nonstick skillet or wok over medium-high heat. Add 2 tablespoons water and the seasonings. Stir-fry for 15 seconds. Add the sauce, cover, and steam for 3 minutes.

3. When the eggplant is done, transfer it to a warming platter and pour the sauce over the eggplant. Warm in oven for 5 to 10 minutes before serving.

* You can purchase Oriental eggplant at health food stores, Asian markets, or better supermarkets. Oriental eggplant should not be peeled, but if you use regular eggplant, peel it because the skin has a bitter taste.

Amount Per Serving

Calories 59   Calories from Fat 3   Total Calories From: Fat 5% Protein 14% Carb. 81%

Vitamin A 2%   Vitamin C 6%   Iron 6%

Tongue-Tickling Curried Greens

I like to serve these greens alongside a platter of Country-Style Tofu Sausage (see page 177).

6 SERVINGS

extra-virgin olive oil cooking spray

1 small sweet onion, diced

3 cloves garlic, finely minced

1 cup red potatoes, diced

1 carrot, sliced

1 cup Basic Vegetable Stock (see page 78)

2 teaspoons curry powder

1 teaspoon sea salt or salt substitute

1 teaspoon black pepper

½ pound turnip greens, coarsely chopped

½ pound curly kale, coarsely chopped

1 tablespoon arrowroot, dissolved in a little water

1. Heat a nonstick soup pot that has been sprayed with olive oil cooking spray. Sauté onion and garlic until onion is translucent. Add potatoes, carrots, and stock. Cover and simmer until potatoes are tender.

2. Stir in curry, salt, and pepper, mixing well. Add turnip greens and kale. Cook until greens are bright green and tender.

3. Add arrowroot and simmer until sauce begins to thicken. Remove from heat and serve.

Amount Per Serving

Calories 76   Calories from Fat 10   Total Calories From: Fat 13% Protein 10% Carb. 77%

Vitamin A 59%   Vitamin C 49%   Iron 7%

Swiss Chard with Tomatoes

Similar to spinach, Swiss chard has a stronger flavor and is equally delicious with all sorts of entrées.

4 SERVINGS

2 bunches Swiss chard, washed and sliced into 1-inch wide ribbons, stems removed and diced

extra-virgin olive oil cooking spray

1 small onion, finely diced

2 cloves garlic, finely minced

1 cup Basic Vegetable Stock (see page 78) or water

½ cup cilantro, chopped

2 tomatoes, seeded and finely diced

sea salt or salt substitute, to taste

freshly milled black pepper, to taste

1. Cook the reserved chard stems in boiling water for about 10 minutes or steam until tender. Set aside.

2. Heat a large nonstick skillet or wok and spray it with extra-virgin olive oil cooking spray. Sauté the onion, stirring occasionally until it softens (about 5 minutes). Add the garlic and sauté an additional 30 seconds.

3. Add the chard, ¼ cup of the vegetable stock, cilantro, salt, and pepper. Cover tightly and cook over low heat for 45 minutes. Check occasionally to make sure there's enough moisture. If anything is sticking, add more broth as needed.

4. Add the cooked chard stems, remaining vegetable broth, and tomatoes. Continue to cook for another minute or so to warm through. Serve hot.

Amount Per Serving

Calories 52   Calories from Fat 8   Total Calories From: Fat 14% Protein 12% Carb. 74%

Vitamin A 26%   Vitamin C 44%   Iron 5%

Buffy's Delicious Greens

Greens are one of those simply delicious, really nutritious side dishes often overlooked. We love them steamed, curried, fresh in salads, or most any way. But to go along with those black-eyed peas, this is our favorite!

8 SERVINGS

3 pounds collard greens, or substitute other greens such as mustard, Swiss chard, spinach, or kale

extra-virgin olive oil spray

1 onion, chopped

2 cloves garlic, minced

1 red bell pepper, chopped

1 quart Basic Vegetable Stock (see page 78)

2 teaspoons brown sugar

1 tablespoon cider vinegar

sea salt or salt substitute, to taste

freshly milled black pepper, to taste

1. Discard tough stems and yellowed leaves from greens. Rinse well and drain. If you use spinach, keep it separate from the other greens.

2. Heat a nonstick skillet or wok over medium heat. Spray it with extra-virgin olive oil spray. Sauté onion, garlic, and bell pepper, stirring often, for 5 minutes or until the onions become translucent. Stir in stock, sugar, and vinegar, then add the greens (except spinach). Add salt and pepper to taste.

3. Cover. Bring to a boil over high heat. Lower heat and simmer, stirring occasionally, until greens are tender when pierced, about 45 minutes (if using spinach, stir in after 20 minutes).

Amount Per Serving

Calories 99   Calories from Fat 13   Total Calories From: Fat 13% Protein 12% Carb. 75%

Vitamin A 126%   Vitamin C 98%   Iron 4%

Seattle's Best Creamed Greens

Full of complex flavors and pleasing to the eye, this is a delightful dish.

8 SERVINGS

1 cup water or Basic Vegetable Stock (see page 78)

2 medium red potatoes (unpeeled), coarsely chopped

1 onion, coarsely chopped

1 12-ounce package low-fat silken tofu

3 cups nonfat soy or rice milk

3 to 4 sweet bell peppers of different colors, coarsely chopped

1 mild-hot pepper, finely chopped (optional)

3 cloves garlic, minced

1 pound greens (spinach, mustard, collard, Swiss chard, watercress), coarsely chopped

sea salt or salt substitute, to taste

freshly milled black pepper, to taste

1. Cook potatoes and onions in water in large saucepan or skillet just until water is absorbed. Be careful not to let potatoes burn.

2. Blend tofu and 1 cup milk in blender until creamy.

3. Add tofu mixture, peppers, garlic, and greens to potato mixture. Gradually add more milk until desired consistency is reached. Season with salt and pepper. Simmer for an additional 5 minutes or so and serve.

Amount Per Serving

Calories 101   Calories from Fat 19   Total Calories From: Fat 19% Protein 20% Carb. 61%

Vitamin A 1%   Vitamin C 16%   Iron 17%

No-Cream Creamed Spinach

You'll never miss the dairy in this flavorful side dish. Substitute other leafy greens for the spinach to add variety.

6 SERVINGS

2 tablespoons cornstarch

1 cup plain nonfat soymilk

4 cups spinach, well rinsed and trimmed, or 2 10-ounce bags washed spinach

extra-virgin olive oil spray

1 onion, thinly sliced

¼ cup low-fat silken tofu (2 ounces)

2 teaspoons granulated onion

½ teaspoon brewer's yeast flakes

¼ teaspoon freshly grated nutmeg, or ground nutmeg

⅛ teaspoon sea salt or salt substitute

white pepper, to taste (optional)

1. Put a large pot of water over high heat and bring to a boil.

2. Meanwhile, place cornstarch in a small saucepan. Slowly pour in soymilk, stirring constantly to blend. Set over medium heat and bring to a boil. Continue stirring constantly and cook until sauce is thick, about 10 minutes. Remove from heat and set aside.

3. Blanch spinach for 1 minute in prepared pot of boiling water. Drain immediately and press out excess liquid.

4. Spray a sauté pan with cooking spray and cook thinly sliced raw onion over low heat until light brown, about 10 minutes. Set aside.

5. Place spinach, onion, tofu, granulated onion, brewer's yeast, and nutmeg in a food processor or blender. Process thoroughly.

6. In a saucepan combine spinach mixture and cream sauce. Cook over low heat, stirring occasionally, until hot. Season with salt and add white pepper if desired.

Amount Per Serving

Calories 49   Calories from Fat 9   Total Calories From: Fat 18% Protein 21% Carb. 61%

Vitamin A 50%   Vitamin C 21%   Iron 7%

Cauliflower in Curry Sauce

If you wish to vary this dish, add broccoli florets along with the cauliflower. It's a great combination!

6 SERVINGS

2 cloves garlic, minced

1 pound tomatoes, chopped

⅓ cup water

1 teaspoon curry powder

½ teaspoon turmeric

½ teaspoon ground cumin

2 cloves garlic, minced

1⁄16 teaspoon ground cinnamon

1 bay leaf

4 cups cauliflower florets

4 ounces low-fat silken tofu

brown rice, cooked

1. Sauté the garlic for 30 seconds in a large nonstick skillet or wok. Next combine tomatoes, water, and spices. Bring to a boil over medium-low heat. Cover and simmer 5 minutes, stirring occasionally. Reserve ½ cup liquid.

2. Add cauliflower. Cover and cook for 10 minutes, or until cauliflower is crunchy-tender. Stir occasionally.

3. Blend the reserved liquid and tofu in a blender until smooth. Add to the cauliflower mixture and blend until heated through but do not boil.

4. Remove from heat, discard bay leaf, and serve with brown rice.

Amount Per Serving

Calories 44   Calories from Fat 5   Total Calories From: Fat 10% Protein 20% Carb. 70%

Vitamin A 10%   Vitamin C 113%   Iron 7%

Broccoli Garlic Stir-Fry

With the addition of hoisin sauce and black bean sauce, this dish takes on a sinfully rich taste. It will soon become one of your favorites.

4 SERVINGS

extra-virgin olive oil spray

10 cloves garlic,
coarsely chopped

¼ cup Basic Vegetable Stock
(see page 78)

¼ teaspoon black bean sauce
(see glossary)

2 teaspoons hoisin sauce
(see glossary)

1 yellow bell pepper, broiled, skinned,
and cut into thin slivers

1 red bell pepper, broiled,
skinned, and cut into thin slivers

4 cups broccoli florets

sea salt or salt substitute, to taste

freshly milled black pepper, to taste

egg white of one hard boiled egg

1. In a large nonstick skillet or wok sprayed with extra-virgin olive oil spray, sauté the garlic until lightly browned, about 30 seconds.

2. Add the vegetable stock, black bean sauce, hoisin sauce, bell peppers, and broccoli. Bring to a boil. Reduce heat. Simmer, covered, about 3-5 minutes, or until the broccoli is crunchy-tender.

3. Put broccoli with sauce into a warmed serving dish. Coarsely chop the boiled egg white and sprinkle over top of the dish. Serve immediately.

Amount Per Serving

Calories 56   Calories from Fat 5   Total Calories From: Fat 8% Protein 24% Carb. 68%

Vitamin A 49%   Vitamin C 199%   Iron 6%

Tempeh Pepper Steak

This mouth-watering tempeh recipe is easy to make. Serve with brown rice and Stir-Fry Greens (see page 163) for a bountiful meal.

4 SERVINGS

¼ cup tamari soy sauce

4 cloves garlic, minced

1 onion, diced

2 8-ounce packages grain tempeh

2 red or green bell peppers, diced

2 onions, thinly sliced

1 cup tomato puree

¼ cup water

2 bay leaves

¼ cup celery, diced

1 tablespoon fresh thyme, chopped

2 tablespoons fresh parsley, chopped

1. Mix the first 3 ingredients. Cut tempeh into steaks each approximately ½ inch thick. Pour half the soy sauce mixture in the bottom of a 9 x 13-inch dish. Arrange tempeh steaks over marinade and pour the remainder on top of each slice. Allow tempeh steaks to marinate for a minimum of 2 hours.

2. One-half hour before serving, sauté tempeh steaks in a nonstick skillet until brown on both sides. Remove from skillet and set aside.

3. Simmer all remaining ingredients in the same nonstick pan for 5 minutes. Return tempeh steaks and the marinade to the pan and simmer slowly for an additional 15 minutes.

4. Serve tempeh steaks with the vegetables and sauce.

Amount Per Serving

Calories 179   Calories from Fat 29   Total Calories From: Fat 16% Protein 22% Carb. 62%

Vitamin A 63%   Vitamin C 175%   Iron 31%

Country-Style Tofu Sausage

These delicious vegetarian patties make a great breakfast treat! It's best to mix the ingredients the night before you plan to cook them.

6 SERVINGS

1 pound tofu,
which has been frozen and thawed*

1 onion, finely minced

1 slice whole-grain bread, crumbled

3 cloves garlic, finely minced or grated

3 tablespoons fresh parsley,
finely minced

2 tablespoons fresh sage, finely minced

1 tablespoon fresh marjoram,
finely minced

¼ teaspoon chili powder

2 teaspoons nutritional yeast**

2 tablespoons tamari soy sauce

⅓ teaspoon black pepper

1 Granny Smith apple,
peeled and grated

1 tablespoon egg substitute,
to bind mixture

1. Crumble tofu with fingers. Add all other ingredients and mix thoroughly with hands.

2. Form patties and cook in medium-hot nonstick skillet, a few minutes on each side.

*You can freeze tofu in an unopened tub. Thaw, then squeeze to remove all liquid. Frozen tofu takes on a spongy texture that gives body to this dish.

**Nutritional yeast, not to be confused with brewer's yeast, consists of delicious flakes that add a rich, cheese-like flavor and creaminess to a dish.

Amount Per Serving

Calories 114	Calories from Fat 35	Total Calories From: Fat 31% Protein 26% Carb. 43%
		Vitamin A 4% Vitamin C 42% Iron 26%

Penne with Herb Tomato Sauce

In the winter when all those fresh juicy tomatoes have been dehydrated, this very simple sauce is delicious on all types of pasta.

4 SERVINGS

⅓ cup sun-dried tomatoes

¾ cup boiling water

2 teaspoons extra-virgin olive oil

1 cup onion, diced

4 cloves garlic, minced

pinch of sugar

1 28-ounce can whole plum tomatoes

1 bay leaf

1 teaspoon fresh thyme leaves, chopped

1½ teaspoons orange zest, minced

10 ounces penne pasta

¼ cup chopped fresh basil leaves, for garnish

1. Combine sun-dried tomatoes and boiling water. Set aside for 15 minutes.

2. Heat oil over medium heat in a large nonstick skillet. Add onion and cook 7 minutes or until onions are translucent. Add garlic and cook 1 minute more.

3. Stir in sun-dried tomatoes along with water, sugar, plum tomatoes with juice, bay leaf, thyme, and orange zest. Bring mixture to a boil. Reduce heat to low and simmer until thickened, about 15 minutes.

4. Cook pasta according to package directions. Drain, reserving ½ cup cooking liquid. Add reserved cooking liquid back into drained pasta.

5. Divide pasta among four serving plates. Remove bay leaf from sauce and spoon the sauce over the pasta. Garnish with fresh basil and serve.

Amount Per Serving

Calories 368   Calories from Fat 48   Total Calories From: Fat 13% Protein 13% Carb. 74%

Vitamin A 28%   Vitamin C 79%   Iron 14%

Japanese Noodles in the Green

We have hosted many students from Japan over the years, and this dish is always a hit!

4 SERVINGS

2 ½ ounces thin rice-stick noodles

1 ½ cups Basic Vegetable Stock
(see page 78)

1 ½ teaspoons dried sage

1 teaspoon tamari soy sauce

3 cloves garlic, minced

¼ cup sweet red bell pepper, diced

3 cups spinach, shredded

1 cup green onion, minced

1. In a large pot of boiling water, cook the noodles for 4 minutes. Drain and set aside.

2. In a large nonstick skillet or wok, combine the stock, sage, soy sauce, garlic, and bell pepper. Bring the mixture to a simmer.

3. Add the noodles. Do not stir or the noodles will tangle; instead gently move them around using chopsticks or tongs. When the noodles are heated, add the spinach and scallions. Simmer 15-20 seconds, or until the spinach is wilted. Serve in shallow bowls.

Amount Per Serving

Calories 102   Calories from Fat 13   Total Calories From: Fat 12% Protein 19% Carb. 69%

Vitamin A 59%   Vitamin C 29%   Iron 14%

Savory Rice Pilaf

Serve with Basic Oven-Roasted Vegetables (see page 157) and finish with a fresh fruit platter for a very satisfying meal.

6 SERVINGS

2 cups brown rice, uncooked

1 large onion, diced

3½ cups Basic Vegetable Stock
(see page 78) or water

½ cup unsweetened apple juice

2 cloves garlic, minced

2 teaspoons lemon juice

½ teaspoon dried thyme

¼ cup steamed edamame
(fresh or frozen whole soybeans),
optional

1. In a 2-quart nonstick saucepan, combine the rice and onion. Stir over medium heat until the rice is golden brown, about 5 minutes

2. Add the stock, apple juice, garlic, lemon juice, and thyme. Bring to a boil. Reduce the heat to low, cover the pan, and simmer until all the liquid has been absorbed and the rice is tender, about 40 minutes. Add the edamame at this time, if desired.

3. Fluff with a fork before serving.

Amount Per Serving

Calories 283   Calories from Fat 28   Total Calories From: Fat 6% Protein 8% Carb. 86%

Vitamin A 0%   Vitamin C 22%   Iron 18%

Basque Spanish Rice

I often make this dish with leftover rice for one of our favorite quick meal dishes. I simply sauté the onions, bell peppers, garlic, and tomatoes and add the cooked rice and seasoning to the mixture. It's fast, easy, and delicious.

4 SERVINGS

1 cup onion, diced

½ cup red or green bell pepper, diced

¼ teaspoon cayenne pepper, or more if you like it hot

2 cloves garlic, minced

3 to 4 tomatoes, diced

1¼ cups long-grain brown rice

sea salt or salt substitute, to taste

freshly milled black pepper, to taste

2 cups boiling water

parsley, for garnish

1. Sauté onion, bell pepper, cayenne, and garlic, uncovered, until brown, in a large nonstick skillet that has a tight-fitting lid.

2. Mix in tomatoes and water and bring to a boil. Stir in rice and cover pan. Lower heat and cook until water is absorbed, approximately 45 minutes. Check seasoning and adjust to taste.

Amount Per Serving

Calories 257   Calories from Fat 19   Total Calories From: Fat 7% Protein 10% Carb. 83%

Vitamin A 23%   Vitamin C 74%   Iron 8%

Condiments, Sauces,

and Spices

▼

Condiments, sauces, and spices enhance and "dress up" many foods, from snacks to main dishes. Many commercially prepared products such as the condiments and sauces you buy at the grocery store are often high in the wrong kinds of fat and low in nutritional value. By making your own, you can be sure of what you're actually adding to your favorite foods. Many people have never thought about making their own mayonnaise, chutney, or marinades from scratch. These simple, delicious recipes let you skip right from thinking to doing … and enjoying!

Fresh Herbs Made Easy

Fresh herbs offer a wonderful way to enhance any dish or meal. A sprig or sprinkling of fresh herbs can add an amazing amount of fragrance, appearance, and flavor. Put a tray of herbs on the table during meals so each person can tear off bits of basil leaves, cilantro, tarragon, Italian parsley, or whatever herbs he or she likes. This allows each person to season rice, beans, salads, and other dishes to suit individual taste.

Nippy Bean Dips and Spreads

Beans make a great alternative to cheese spreads and sour cream dips. The basic directions are the same for all the bean dips:

- *If using your own beans, make sure they're very soft and mash easily. Drain beans but save at least ½ cup of the liquid.*
- *If using canned beans, drain, reserving the liquid, and rinse beans in a strainer under cold water to remove excess sodium.*
- *Transfer the beans to a blender and blend them until smooth, adding only enough liquid to facilitate blending.*
- *Stir in the listed condiments and spices.*
- *Serve the spreads on whole-grain crackers, toasted pita chips, fat-free tortilla chips, or crudités (bite-size broccoli, cauliflower, carrots, snow peas, mushrooms, celery, radishes, cucumbers, or other cut fresh vegetables).*

Roasted Garlic Bean Dip/Spread

4 cloves large roasted garlic, chopped (see page 187)

¾ cup white beans, cooked (rinsed and drained if using canned)

1 teaspoon extra-virgin olive oil

sea salt or salt substitute, to taste

Chili Bean Dip/Spread

1 cup white beans, cooked

1 teaspoon chili powder

1 teaspoon onion powder

1 teaspoon green chili peppers, chopped

¼ teaspoon cayenne pepper

Creole Bean Dip/Spread

1 cup kidney beans, cooked

2 tablespoons sweet green bell peppers, finely chopped

2 tablespoons tomatoes, minced

5 drops hot pepper sauce or ½ teaspoon Red Chili Paste (see page 196)

Coriander White Bean Dip/Spread

1 cup white beans, cooked
(rinsed and drained if using canned)

4 cloves garlic, finely minced

1 teaspoon extra-virgin olive oil

1 teaspoon ground cumin

1 teaspoon ground coriander

pinch of salt

pinch of cayenne pepper

Combine all ingredients and blend in blender until smooth.

These dips/spreads may be made 1 day ahead and chilled, covered. Bring to room temperature before serving.

The nutritional content may vary a little with each bean recipe. Below is a general guideline.

Amount Per Serving

Calories 32   Calories from Fat 6   Total Calories From: Fat 19% Protein 20% Carb. 61%

Vitamin A 0%   Vitamin C 1%   Iron 3%

Tofu Spread

1 pound low-fat silken firm tofu

1 tablespoon onion, finely chopped

¼ cup celery, finely chopped

3 tablespoons Buffy's Eggless Mayonnaise (see page 195)

1 tablespoon sweet pickle relish

1 teaspoon Dijon mustard

¼ teaspoon dried dill weed

1 tablespoon dried parsley

sea salt or salt substitute, to taste

freshly milled black pepper, to taste

Red Chili Paste (optional; see page 196)

1. Press the liquid out of the tofu. Mash the tofu coarsely with a fork. Stir in the onion and celery.

2. Combine the remaining ingredients and mix into the tofu.

Amount Per Serving

Calories 105   Calories from Fat 50   Total Calories From: Fat 48% Protein 36% Carb. 16%

Vitamin A 4%   Vitamin C 20%   Iron 36%

Roasted Garlic

I like to bake a dozen or more garlic heads and add the roasted garlic cloves to olive oil, or make a spread for toast. Or, better yet, bake lots and make Centennial Garlic Soup (see page 95) or Nippy Bean Dips and Spreads (see page 184).

3 heads (3 to 4 ounces each) garlic
extra-virgin olive oil

1. About halfway down garlic heads, cut the tough outer skin with a paring knife. Pull off upper half of outer skin to expose cloves. Arrange heads, root ends down, in a close-fitting shallow casserole (6 to 8 inches wide). Drizzle lightly with olive oil.

2. Bake garlic in a 350° F oven until it is very soft when pressed and cut cloves are richly browned, 45 to 55 minutes.

3. Serve hot or at room temperature. Pull cloves from whole heads and squeeze garlic out. Pluck cut cloves from half heads.

To make garlic oil from the roasted garlic, cut 5 large roasted garlic cloves in half, add to 1½ cups olive oil, and cover tightly. Let stand in the refrigerator for at least 15 days. Shake occasionally. Use garlic oil in cooking, as a dip for bread, or in salad dressings.

Amount Per Serving

Calories 7   Calories from Fat 0   Total Calories From: Fat 4% Protein 14% Carb. 82%

Vitamin A 0%   Vitamin C 2%   Iron 0%

Roasted Pumpkin Seed Pesto

This is a delicious and unique pesto that you can use on baked squash or over your favorite pasta, or spread on crackers or crusty bread.

1 cup green pumpkin seeds

3 large cloves garlic, roasted and peeled

1 tablespoon extra-virgin olive oil

1 tablespoon mellow white miso paste (see glossary)

1 tablespoon cilantro

1. Roast green pumpkin seeds at 325° F for 10 minutes.

2. Pulse ingredients in a blender, stopping to scrape down the sides with a rubber spatula between pulses, just until roughly chopped and combined.

3. Taste and adjust seasoning as necessary.

Amount Per Serving

Calories 418   Calories from Fat 233   Total Calories From: Fat 56% Protein 11% Carb. 33%

Vitamin A 1%   Vitamin C 0%   Iron 12%

Tomatillos Chutney

A wonderful aroma will fill your home when you make this chutney. It is refreshing when served with beans or grains.

1 PINT

1 pound fresh tomatillos,* husked, rinsed, and quartered

2 small red bell or pimento peppers, diced

1 green bell pepper, diced

8 green onions including tops, sliced

4 jalapeño peppers, finely diced

⅔ cup balsamic vinegar

3 tablespoons honey

1 tablespoon cilantro, chopped

1 teaspoon sea salt or salt substitute

1 clove garlic, minced

¼ teaspoon cayenne pepper

¼ teaspoon ground cumin

1. Combine all ingredients in large saucepan or stockpot. Bring to a boil, stirring frequently. Reduce heat to low and cook gently until thick, stirring occasionally, for 30 to 35 minutes.

2. Pour into storage jars or attractive serving containers and cool thoroughly, cover and refrigerate. Best used within 5 days, or you can freeze it.

*Tomatillos can be found in the vegetable section of many large supermarkets or at your Mexican market.

Amount Per Serving

Calories 442   Calories from Fat 6   Total Calories From: Fat 3% Protein 6% Carb. 91%

Vitamin A 401%   Vitamin C 844%   Iron 22%

Pickled Cabbage Relish

The flavor and simplicity of this recipe make this a dish you will want to keep around. The recipe given is for 1 pint, but you'll probably want to multiply the yield several times over.

1 PINT

1 cup red cabbage, thinly sliced

½ cup green cabbage, thinly sliced

½ cup onions, thinly sliced

2 tablespoons fresh jalapeño peppers, minced

½ cup distilled white vinegar

½ teaspoon sea salt or salt substitute

1. Mix cabbages, onion, jalapeño peppers, vinegar, and salt in a large bowl. Let stand about 30 minutes.

2. Lift out with a slotted spoon to serve. Store pickled relish (in liquid) in the refrigerator.

Amount Per Serving

Calories 98   Calories from Fat 4   Total Calories From: Fat 4% Protein 11% Carb. 85%

Vitamin A 42%   Vitamin C 179%   Iron 5%

Home-Cooked Salsa

We like salsa with scrambled tofu, baked potatoes, lentil dishes, as well as on the traditional burritos and taco dishes.

12 SERVINGS

6 fresh tomatoes or
32 ounces canned, finely chopped

1 tablespoon ground cumin

1 teaspoon ground coriander

½ teaspoon cayenne pepper

½ teaspoon dried or
2 teaspoons fresh oregano,
finely chopped

½ teaspoon dried basil or
2 teaspoons fresh basil,
finely chopped

1 onion, diced

½ teaspoon sea salt or salt substitute

5 cloves garlic, minced

2 green bell peppers, finely chopped

1. If you are using canned tomatoes, pour the tomatoes through a strainer or a colander to drain off some juice. You will need about 2½ cups of mostly drained tomatoes to make a thick salsa (save the juice to use in soup).

2. Mix the spices together.

3. Heat a nonstick skillet and add the onion. Sauté 4 minutes, adding water as needed to prevent burning. Add the garlic and cook an additional minute. Reduce the heat and add the spice mixture. Sauté for 30 seconds to enhance the flavors, stirring constantly so nothing sticks and burns.

4. Add the tomatoes. Simmer fresh tomatoes for 15 minutes (canned for 5 minutes). Add the salt and green peppers and simmer for 5 minutes longer.

5. If necessary, add more seasoning. If you like hotter salsa, add more cayenne pepper.

The salsa keeps nicely for about a week in the refrigerator, or for as long as you like in the freezer.

Amount Per Serving

Calories 31	Calories from Fat 4	Total Calories From: Fat 11% Protein 14% Carb. 75%
		Vitamin A 10% Vitamin C 48% Iron 4%

Tomato-Basil Dressing

This delicious dressing will keep for about a week in the refrigerator.

12 SERVINGS

6 sun-dried tomatoes

1 cup fresh tomato, coarsely chopped

2 cloves garlic, finely minced

¼ cup fresh basil, coarsely chopped

¼ cup water

2 tablespoons balsamic vinegar

sea salt or salt substitute, to taste

1. Place the sun-dried tomatoes in a heat-proof bowl and cover with boiling water. Set aside.

2. Combine remaining ingredients in a blender or food processor. Drain the softened sun-dried tomatoes and add them to the other ingredients. Purée the mixture until smooth and serve.

Amount Per Serving

Calories 21   Calories from Fat 1   Total Calories From: Fat 4% Protein 11% Carb. 85%

Vitamin A 3%   Vitamin C 8%   Iron 4%

Russian Dressing
with Sun-Dried Tomatoes

A thick and creamy non-dairy, no-egg dressing. Great on sandwiches or greens.

6 sun-dried tomato halves
(not oil-packed)

¼ cup boiling water

5 ounces low-fat silken tofu

2 teaspoons prepared horseradish

1 teaspoon catsup

1 teaspoon shallot or onion, minced

½ teaspoon Worcestershire sauce

sea salt, to taste

freshly milled black pepper, to taste

1. In a small bowl, cover sun-dried tomatoes with boiling water and let sit until tomatoes have softened, 15 to 20 minutes. Remove tomatoes and chop coarsely; reserve soaking liquid.

2. In a blender, combine tomatoes with remaining ingredients. Blend until smooth, stopping to scrape down sides two or three times. Add soaking liquid, as needed, to achieve desired consistency.

Amount Per Serving

Calories 6   Calories from Fat 0   Total Calories From: Fat 18% Protein 5% Carb. 77%

Vitamin A 1%   Vitamin C 2%   Iron 0%

Orange-Soy Dressing

Sinfully delicious! You can use this dressing for your steamed vegetables and as a dressing over your favorite salad. I try to keep this made up in my refrigerator at all times.

12 SERVINGS

½ cup freshly squeezed orange juice

1 tablespoon maple syrup

3 tablespoons tamari soy sauce

¼ cup rice vinegar

4 teaspoons mirin (see glossary)

Combine all ingredients and blend thoroughly. Refrigerate until ready to use.

If you want a thicker consistency to your dressing add ⅛ teaspoon xantham gum, which can be purchased in good health food stores.

Amount Per Serving

Calories 13   Calories from Fat 0   Total Calories From: Fat 2% Protein 16% Carb. 82%

Vitamin A 0%   Vitamin C 6%   Iron 1%

Buffy's Eggless Mayonnaise

Mayonnaise is one of those condiments we have always put on our sandwiches, and used to make potato salad, macaroni salad, and a myriad of other dishes. You will find this tastes just as good as the traditional mayonnaise, but has the benefits of soy.

1 8-ounce package silken tofu

2 tablespoons soymilk

1 tablespoon brown rice vinegar

1 tablespoon lemon juice

1 tablespoon mellow white miso (see glossary)

1 tablespoon Dijon mustard

¾ teaspoon sugar

Place all ingredients in a blender and blend until smooth. Refrigerate overnight before using. Keeps refrigerated for 2-3 days (if it separates, just reblend).

Amount Per Serving

Calories 9   Calories from Fat 4   Total Calories From: Fat 66% Protein 26% Carb. 8%

Vitamin A 0%   Vitamin C 0%   Iron 2%

Red Chili Paste

Inspired by Thai cooking, you can use this chili paste whenever you wish to add some heat to your food. Because chili peppers vary in size and flavor, adjust the amount as you see fit. This creation is hot, garlicky, and bold.

16 small dried red chili peppers

2 shallots, finely chopped

10 cloves garlic, finely minced

2 tablespoons fresh galangal
(see glossary)

2 stalks lemongrass

1 teaspoon white peppercorns

½ teaspoon coriander seeds

2 coriander roots

1 to 2 tablespoons water

1. Soak chili peppers covered in water about 1 hour or until just softened. Drain and discard water.

2. In a food processor, blend chilies, shallots, garlic, galangal, lemongrass, peppercorns, coriander seeds, and coriander roots until smooth. Gradually add 1 to 2 tablespoons water to assist in the blending. The paste should be smooth, but not wet.

3. Store in an airtight container in the refrigerator for 1 to 2 weeks, or freeze up to 6 months.

Amount Per Serving

Calories 66   Calories from Fat 3   Total Calories From: Fat 5% Protein 15% Carb. 80%

Vitamin A 25%   Vitamin C 17%   Iron 6%

Thai Marinade

Use this to marinate vegetables, tempeh, or tofu for a wonderful taste sensation!

8 SERVINGS

½ cup lime juice

½ cup lemon juice

½ cup cilantro, minced

2 teaspoons tamari soy sauce

1 teaspoon ginger root,
peeled and grated

1 teaspoon Red Chili Paste
(see page 196)

8 cloves garlic, finely minced

In a small bowl, mix all the ingredients in the order listed.

*Marinate vegetables, tempeh, or tofu for at least 1 hour. Broil or grill. Garnish tempeh or tofu with cilantro and green onions.

Amount Per Serving

Calories 12   Calories from Fat 0   Total Calories From: Fat 2% Protein 12% Carb. 86%

Vitamin A 1%   Vitamin C 14%   Iron 1%

Lime Marinade

Marinate vegetables, tofu, or tempeh with this marinade* and use as a dressing on fruit salad such as papaya, oranges, raspberries, and blueberries.

6 SERVINGS

½ cup fresh lime juice

½ teaspoon lime peel, finely minced

2 tablespoons fresh cilantro, minced

2 green jalapeño chilies, stemmed, seeded, and minced

2 teaspoons sugar

Mix all ingredients together until well blended.

*When marinating vegetables, marinate at least 8 hours or overnight. Grill or broil as desired.

Amount Per Serving

Calories 16   Calories from Fat 1   Total Calories From: Fat 4% Protein 10% Carb. 86%

Vitamin A 0%   Vitamin C 12%   Iron 1%

Jamaican Marinade

This is a great marinade for tofu squares, tempeh steaks, or baked vegetables.*

8 SERVINGS

4 fresh green chili peppers
or 2 teaspoons Red Chili Paste
(see page 196)

¾ cup onions, coarsely chopped

3 tablespoons tamari soy sauce

¼ cup balsamic vinegar

2 tablespoons brown sugar

3 teaspoons ginger root,
peeled and grated

3 cloves garlic, finely minced

1 teaspoon dried thyme

1 teaspoon dried oregano

1 teaspoon ground allspice

1 teaspoon ground cloves

1 teaspoon ground cinnamon

¾ teaspoon freshly milled black pepper

½ teaspoon ground ginger

Combine all ingredients in a blender or food processor and purée until smooth.

*Marinate pressed tofu squares, tempeh steaks, or root vegetables for a minimum of 2 hours.
Bake in preheated 400° F oven.

Amount Per Serving

Calories 25   Calories from Fat 1   Total Calories From: Fat 5% Protein 11% Carb. 84%

Vitamin A 0%   Vitamin C 3%   Iron 4%

Ginger-Soy Marinade

3 green onions, including tops, finely chopped

2½ tablespoons tamari soy sauce

1 tablespoon ginger root, peeled and grated

⅓ cup orange juice concentrate

⅓ cup apple cider vinegar

2½ tablespoons lemon juice, freshly squeezed

2 cloves garlic, finely minced

In a small bowl mix all the ingredients in the order listed. Marinate your favorite vegetables, tempeh steaks, or tofu squares at least 6 hours or overnight. Broil or grill.

Amount Per Serving

Calories 35   Calories from Fat 0   Total Calories From: Fat 1% Protein 10% Carb. 89%

Vitamin A 1%   Vitamin C 37%   Iron 2%

Caribbean Marinade

This marinade is great for baked root vegetables, tempeh, or tofu steaks. Toss vegetables, tempeh, or tofu steaks with the marinade and bake on baking tray at 425° F, stirring occasionally.

1 teaspoon Red Chili Paste

2 cloves garlic, finely minced

2 teaspoons ginger root, peeled and freshly grated

½ teaspoon ground cinnamon

½ teaspoon ground cloves

½ teaspoon ground allspice

½ teaspoon dried thyme

½ teaspoon freshly milled black pepper

1 medium onion, coarsely chopped

1 tablespoon brown sugar, firmly packed

2 tablespoons balsamic vinegar

1 teaspoon extra-virgin olive oil

3 tablespoons tamari soy sauce

Toss all ingredients into blender and purée until smooth. Refrigerate for up to a week.

Amount Per Serving

Calories 99   Calories from Fat 2   Total Calories From: Fat 2% Protein 17% Carb. 81%

Vitamin A 97%   Vitamin C 185%   Iron 16%

Roasted Tomato-Garlic Sauce

I like to double this recipe and freeze it in ice cube trays, then transfer the cubes to resealable bags. It's great to have on hand for adding punch to purchased tomato sauces for those quick meals when I don't have time to make sauce from scratch.

1 CUP

1 cup onion, diced

1 teaspoon extra-virgin olive oil

25 cloves garlic
(approximately 3 heads)

5 tomatoes, cut into 8 wedges

½ cup water

1 tablespoon balsamic vinegar

½ teaspoon sea salt or salt substitute

1. Preheat oven to 450° F.

2. Combine onion, olive oil, garlic, and tomatoes in a 13 x 9-inch baking dish. Bake at 450° F for 20 minutes.

3. Combine tomato mixture, water, vinegar, and salt in a large saucepan and bring to a boil. Cook over high heat for 10 minutes.

4. Place in a blender or food processor and blend until desired consistency.

Amount Per Serving

Calories 39   Calories from Fat 7   Total Calories From: Fat 18% Protein 12% Carb. 70%

Vitamin A 8%   Vitamin C 32%   Iron 2%

Vietnamese Dipping Sauce

We use this wonderful dipping sauce with rolled-up rice papers filled with vegetables. It's absolutely yummy!

3 tablespoons warm water

3 tablespoons sugar

3 tablespoons lemon juice
or rice vinegar

6 tablespoons fish sauce
(see glossary)

1 clove garlic, finely chopped

2 teaspoons hot chili peppers

Dissolve sugar in warm water and add remaining ingredients. Mix thoroughly.

Amount Per Serving

Calories 287   Calories from Fat 14   Total Calories From: Fat 5% Protein 8% Carb. 87%

Vitamin A 7%   Vitamin C 37%   Iron 20%

Stir-Fry Sauce

We often make stir-fry vegetables at our home. The recipe is quick, easy, and delicious, and we enjoy the crunchiness of the vegetables.

½ cup orange juice or pineapple juice

¼ cup tamari soy sauce

1 tablespoon ginger root,
peeled and grated

3 cloves garlic, minced

1½ tablespoons honey

½ teaspoon sesame oil

2 tablespoons cornstarch

Mix all ingredients in a blender and use with your favorite low-fat stir-fry recipe. This mixture will keep for about a week in the refrigerator.

Amount Per Serving

Calories 71   Calories from Fat 6   Total Calories From: Fat 8% Protein 11% Carb. 81%

Vitamin A 1%   Vitamin C 210%   Iron 3%

Ginger-Garlic Sauce

This sauce is great drizzled over steamed vegetables such as broccoli and cauliflower.

extra-virgin olive oil cooking spray

3 tablespoons ginger root, peeled and freshly grated

2 cloves garlic, minced

1 tablespoon whole wheat flour

1 cup nonfat soymilk

sea salt or salt substitute, to taste

freshly ground black pepper, to taste

1. Spray nonstick saucepan with extra-virgin olive oil. Add garlic and ginger root and cook, stirring often, until golden, about 1 minute. Reduce heat to low.

2. Stir in flour and cook 2 to 3 minutes, stirring constantly to prevent browning. Gradually stir in soymilk, salt, and pepper and cook, stirring frequently, until sauce is thick and bubbly (3 to 5 minutes).

Amount Per Serving

Calories 37   Calories from Fat 2   Total Calories From: Fat 4% Protein 15% Carb. 81%

Vitamin A 0%   Vitamin C 3%   Iron 2%

Original Indian Curry Sauce

A great sauce to serve over steamed vegetables such as carrots or cauliflower.

4 SERVINGS

1 cup onion, finely chopped

3 cloves garlic, finely minced

1 teaspoon extra-virgin olive oil

1 teaspoon ground cumin

½ teaspoon ground coriander

½ teaspoon turmeric

pinch of cayenne pepper

1 cup nonfat soy yogurt

sea salt or salt substitute, to taste

freshly milled black pepper, to taste

1. Heat a nonstick pan over medium-high heat. Add olive oil and sauté onions until nicely browned. Add garlic and a little water as needed to prevent sticking. Sauté an additional minute. Add cumin, coriander, turmeric, and cayenne, and cook, stirring constantly for 2 minutes.

2. Transfer to a blender, add yogurt, and purée until smooth. Add salt and pepper to taste. Transfer to a bowl and serve.

Amount Per Serving

Calories 23   Calories from Fat 2   Total Calories From: Fat 8% Protein 13% Carb. 79%

Vitamin A 0%   Vitamin C 6%   Iron 3%

Herbes de Provence

¼ cup savory, fresh or dried

¼ cup thyme, fresh or dried

¼ cup fennel, fresh or dried

2 teaspoons lavender flowers

½ cup basil, fresh or dried

Combine the herbs and store them in a dark jar until ready to use.

Amount Per Serving

Calories 4   Calories from Fat 1   Total Calories From: Fat 16% Protein 12% Carb. 72%

Vitamin A 1%   Vitamin C 1%   Iron 6%

Breads and Muffins

▼

Most commercially prepared breads, muffins, and baked goods are quite high in dietary fat, making them unsuitable as a regular part of your diet. Sometimes, however, you can't escape the need for something to hold the contents of your sandwich or accompany a nutritious bowl of soup. These recipes feature low-fat alternatives to help you stay on track with your nutrition plan. They are also high in fiber and carbohydrates, giving your body needed energy. Because they feature whole grains and flavorful ingredients, these breads and muffins are sure to add great taste and texture to any meal.

Use Mashed Fruits in Baked Goods Instead of Eggs

Use ¼ cup mashed banana, applesauce, or puréed prunes to replace one egg in a muffin recipe. You'll cut fat and add flavor and texture. Add an extra ½ teaspoon of baking powder, too, to help your muffins bake lighter.

Focaccia Bread

This is an easy-to-prepare flatbread. I often vary this recipe by substituting olives for the sun-dried tomatoes, or adding fresh basil instead of rosemary. Try your own combinations. It's fun to experiment.

8 SERVINGS

3 cups unbleached white flour

¾ cup organic spelt flour*

¼ cup bran flakes

2 teaspoons sea salt or salt substitute

2 packages quick-rise active dry yeast

1 tablespoon extra-virgin olive oil

¼ cup low-fat silken tofu

3 roasted garlic cloves, finely minced

½ cup sun-dried tomatoes, diced

2 tablespoons fresh rosemary, finely minced

extra-virgin olive oil cooking spray

1. Place flours, bran, salt, yeast, olive oil, tofu, garlic, sun-dried tomatoes, and rosemary in a large mixing bowl and stir to mix ingredients. Add 1¾ cups hot water and stir well with large spoon. If dough seems too dry, add a bit more hot water until it forms a ball.

2. Flour breadboard with additional flour, turn dough out onto breadboard and knead for 6 to 8 minutes. Add sprinkles of flour if the dough is sticky under your hands. Form the dough into a ball.

3. Place the dough into a bowl that has been lightly rubbed with olive oil. Cover with a clean cloth and let the dough rise in a warm place for at least 45 minutes.

4. Flatten the dough onto a nonstick cookie sheet until it is ¼ inch thick, cover dough with a clean cloth, and let it rest in a warm place until puffed, approximately 25 minutes.

5. Preheat the oven to 450° F.

6. Lightly spray the bread with the olive oil spray, and bake for 12 to 15 minutes until lightly browned and puffy. Remove from oven. Slice into desired size servings, and serve warm.

*Spelt flour can be purchased at most health food stores.

Amount Per Serving

Calories 209	Calories from Fat 32	Total Calories From: Fat 15% Protein 11% Carb. 74%
		Vitamin A 0% Vitamin C 2% Iron 6%

Homemade Tortillas

When I was growing up on a farm, my father hired many workers from Mexico. They made and ate delicious tortillas daily, and they taught me how to make them. However, the tortillas were loaded with fat. This recipe has that same great taste, without all the fat.

8 SERVINGS

1 cup unbleached white flour

1 cup whole wheat flour

½ teaspoon sea salt or salt substitute

1 teaspoon extra-virgin olive oil

¾ cup nonfat soymilk

1. Sift the flours and salt in a large bowl. Slowly add the oil and just enough soymilk to make a soft dough.

2. If dough is sticky, add a little more flour. Knead a few minutes, cover with a towel, and let sit for 20 minutes.

3. Divide dough into 8 balls. Roll each ball into a thin circle about 10 inches in diameter. While you are rolling, keep dough and tortillas covered with a damp towel so they do not dry out.

4. Cook on a nonstick griddle on medium-high heat until done. Serve hot.

Amount Per Serving

Calories 116   Calories from Fat 10   Total Calories From: Fat 8% Protein 13% Carb. 79%

Vitamin A 0%   Vitamin C 0%   Iron 4%

Maple-Oatmeal Bread

Thanks to the oatmeal, this loaf has an interesting texture, and thanks to the syrup and raisins, it has a light sweetness in taste.

8 SERVINGS

1 cup sifted unbleached white flour

1 cup sifted rye flour

1 teaspoon baking powder

1 teaspoon baking soda

1 teaspoon sea salt or salt substitute

1 cup rolled oats

¾ cup maple syrup

1 cup nonfat soymilk

¼ cup low-fat silken tofu

1 cup raisins

1. Combine flours and sift them together with baking powder, baking soda, and salt. Stir in the oats.

2. Gradually add maple syrup, soymilk, and tofu until mixture is smooth. Stir in the raisins. Pour into a nonstick 9 by 5-inch loaf pan. Let rest at room temperature for 25 minutes.

3. Bake in a moderate 350° F oven for 1 hour. Let cool before slicing.

Amount Per Serving

Calories 290	Calories from Fat 13	Total Calories From: Fat 5% Protein 7% Carb. 88%
		Vitamin A 0% Vitamin C 1% Iron 11%

Whole Wheat Baguettes

The exceptional flavor of this bread is derived from the fresh herbes de Provence. It's delicious toasted, served with your favorite fat-free spread.

16 SERVINGS

1½ cups bread flour
or unbleached white flour

1½ cups whole wheat flour

1 package dry yeast

1 teaspoon salt or salt substitute

¾ cup hot water (120° - 130° F)

¼ cup orange Curaçao

½ cup fresh or 2 tablespoons dried
herbes de Provence (see page 207)

1. Sift and blend the flours together. Measure 1½ cups flour into a mixing bowl and stir in the yeast and salt. Pour in the hot water and the Curaçao. Beat into a smooth batter with a wooden spoon or in the mixer with the flat beater. Stir in the herbes de Provence.

2. Add remaining flour, a small portion at a time, until the batter becomes a mass that can be lifted from the bowl to the work surface or placed under the dough hook.

3. Knead with a rhythmic push-turn fold, using a dough blade or scraper to help in the work. Occasionally throw the dough down against the work surface to speed the kneading process. Knead by hand for about 8 minutes until the ball of dough is smooth and elastic. Add sprinkles of flour to control stickiness.

4. Place the dough in a lightly greased bowl, cover with plastic wrap, and leave at room temperature until it has doubled in bulk, about 50 minutes.

5. Punch down the raised dough and form a ball. Divide the dough into 2 pieces and roll into slender ropes about 12 inches long and 1½ inches thick. Place in a regular twin baguette pan or on a baking sheet.

6. Cover the loaves loosely with plastic wrap and leave to double in volume, about 40 minutes.

7. Preheat the oven to 375° F 20 minutes before baking.

8. Bake about 30 minutes, or until the loaves are a light golden color. When the loaves seem done, turn the bread over and tap the bottom with a forefinger. It should be hard and sound hollow.

9. Turn onto a metal rack and allow to cool before slicing.

Amount Per Serving

Calories 82   Calories from Fat 3   Total Calories From: Fat 4% Protein 13% Carb. 83%

Vitamin A 0%   Vitamin C 0%   Iron 3%

Sweet Squash Muffins

These are moist, like miniature cakes, and loaded with flavor.

12 SERVINGS

extra-virgin olive oil cooking spray

2 egg whites

¼ cup orange juice

1 tablespoon extra-virgin olive oil

¼ cup nonfat soymilk

¼ cup low-fat silken tofu

1 cup cooked acorn squash, mashed

⅓ cup pitted prunes, chopped

½ cup pears, diced

1 tablespoon baking powder

¼ teaspoon ground ginger

¼ teaspoon ground nutmeg

½ teaspoon ground cinnamon

¼ teaspoon sea salt or salt substitute

⅓ cup whole wheat pastry flour

⅓ cup unbleached white flour

⅓ cup spelt flour*

1. Preheat the oven to 375° F.

2. Spray a nonstick muffin tin with olive oil spray.

3. Combine the wet ingredients, including the squash and fruit. In a separate bowl, sift the dry ingredients.

4. Add the dry ingredients to the wet ingredients, mixing until just blended. Divide the batter into 12 muffin cups. These muffins are dense, so fill the muffin cups higher than you would with other batters.

5. Bake for 30 to 35 minutes or until the muffins separate from the pan and bounce back when lightly tapped.

*Spelt flour can be purchased at most health food stores.

Amount Per Serving

Calories 107   Calories from Fat 15   Total Calories From: Fat 14% Protein 11% Carb. 75%

Vitamin A 3%   Vitamin C 6%   Iron 3%

Pizza Pizzazz

While this is an exceptional pizza dough, we also enjoy making breadsticks or a flatbread with this dough.

6 SERVINGS

Pizza Dough

1 tablespoon yeast

1 cup lukewarm water

1 tablespoon honey

1 tablespoon fresh rosemary, finely minced

16 fresh oregano leaves, finely minced

1 tablespoon fresh thyme leaves, finely minced

5 cloves garlic, finely minced

½ teaspoon sea salt or salt substitute

1 tablespoon extra-virgin olive oil

1½ cups unbleached white flour

1. Combine yeast, ½ cup of lukewarm water, and honey in a large mixing bowl. Gently stir, then set aside. Let rest for 10 minutes while yeast comes to life.

2. Combine minced rosemary, oregano, thyme, and garlic. Add minced herbs, salt, oil, and remaining water to yeast mixture. Add flour a little at a time and mix together with a spoon until it becomes too hard to stir. Transfer to a floured surface and knead until smooth (10-12 minutes). Add more flour to surface when necessary to keep dough from sticking. Place dough in an oiled bowl. Cover and let rest for 30 minutes.

3. To make pizza, preheat oven to 350° F. Roll dough out to desired shape. Bake 10-12 minutes. Remove from oven. Raise oven temperature to 450° F. Combine all of the sauce ingredients in a bowl (see below). Spread the sauce on the crust. Layer on the toppings of your choice (see suggestions below) and bake 12-15 minutes.

continued overleaf

Suggested Sauce

4 cups crushed or strained tomatoes

2 teaspoon fresh oregano

2 teaspoons fresh basil

1 clove garlic, minced

Topping Suggestions

fresh mushrooms, sliced

green bell peppers, chopped

red bell peppers, chopped

sweet onions, chopped

zucchini, sliced

fresh spinach, chopped

water-packed artichoke hearts, sliced

garlic, sliced

Amount Per Serving

Calories 148   Calories from Fat 23   Total Calories From: Fat 16% Protein 9% Carb. 75%

Vitamin A 0%   Vitamin C 1%   Iron 3%

Desserts and Treats

▼

How's your sweet tooth? If you're like most people, it often gets the best of you. The average American consumes about 140 pounds of sugar in various forms over the course of a year. One reason sugar consumption is so high is that this ubiquitous substance appears in many forms in many foods where you might not expect to find it. Some packaged breakfast cereals have four teaspoons or more of sugar in each serving, for example.

Sugar is not all bad, of course. In fact, you couldn't survive without it. Your cells require sugar in the form of glucose to carry out the functions of living. Sugar is abundant in nature, in fresh fruits and vegetables. If you consumed only sugar in its natural forms, your diet would be healthy. But high quantities of processed sugars, such as those common in processed foods, overfill your body's needs. So your body converts the overflow into fat.

Three Cheers for Chocolate!

One fatty acid, stearic acid, appears to kill prostate cancer cells and, as a bonus, lower your risk for heart disease as well. Most surprising of all might be the most common source of this fatty acid: dark chocolate.

Stearic acid is abundant in cocoa butter (though not present at all in fat-free cocoa), and in its highest concentration in dark chocolates that contain cocoa butter as their only fat source. Milk chocolate is still a no-no because of the additional fats it contains.

Manufacturers that produce dark chocolate candy bars that don't contain any milk products include Ghirardelli and Lindt.

While there doesn't seem to be any direct correlation between dietary sugar and prostate cancer, there are numerous studies that link excess body fat with an increased risk of developing prostate cancer and lowered response to treatment once prostate cancer is diagnosed. Reducing dietary sugar makes good sense.

Many people believe they just can't live without candy, cakes, pies, pastries, and other commercial products that soothe their cravings for sweets. If you're one of them, these recipes might just change your mind!

Banana Cherry Jello

This recipe uses the natural jelling agent, agar, to thicken liquid. Agar, a sea vegetable rich in fiber and minerals, thickens at room temperature, unlike gelatin, which must be chilled.

8 SERVINGS

1 quart cherry juice

¼ cup agar flakes (see glossary)

1 pint fresh cherries, pitted

2 bananas

mint leaves, for garnish (optional)

fresh cherries, for garnish (optional)

1. Pour juice in a medium saucepan. Sprinkle agar into juice, add fresh cherries, and bring the mixture to a boil. Lower heat and simmer for 10 minutes until agar flakes are completely dissolved.

2. Slice the bananas and put them in the bottom of the serving dishes. Remove the thickened cherry juice from the heat and pour the mixture over the bananas. Let set at room temperature for about an hour.

3. Serve garnished with a cherry and mint leaf, if desired.

Amount Per Serving

Calories 90   Calories from Fat 1   Total Calories From: Fat 1% Protein 3% Carb. 96%

Vitamin A 8%   Vitamin C 24%   Iron 1%

Creamy Orange-Vanilla Popsicle

This delicious popsicle is only a sample of taste treats that can be created. Let your imagination soar and dream up an endless variety of frozen treats! Popsicle holders can be purchased in the summertime at most stores that carry kitchenware.

2 SERVINGS

¾ cup orange juice

¼ cup nonfat soymilk

1 teaspoon vanilla extract

Blend all ingredients in a blender, pour into popsicle holder, and freeze for 2 to 3 hours.

Amount Per Serving

Calories 47   Calories from Fat 2   Total Calories From: Fat 5% Protein 7% Carb. 88%

Vitamin A 2%   Vitamin C 53%   Iron 1%

Banana-Raspberry Popsicle

Popsicle holders can be purchased in the summertime at most stores that carry kitchenware.

2 SERVINGS

1 banana
½ cup raspberries
⅓ cup water

Blend all ingredients in a blender, pour into popsicle holders, and freeze.

Amount Per Serving

Calories 75	Calories from Fat 4	Total Calories From:	Fat 5%	Protein 5%	Carb. 90%
			Vitamin A 2%	Vitamin C 21%	Iron 2%

Papaya Freeze

Nothing could be simpler to make. A scoop of papaya freeze is a wonderful addition to mild-flavored fruit salads.

4 SERVINGS

1 very ripe papaya (approximately 1½ pounds), peeled, halved, and seeded

1 lemon, cut into 4 wedges

1. Wrap each papaya half in plastic wrap and freeze for approximately 3 hours until solid.

2. Transfer papaya to refrigerator about 1 hour before serving. Meanwhile, chill 4 small serving bowls. Just before serving, unwrap each papaya half and coarsely shred.

3. Spoon shredded papaya into chilled serving bowls. Serve lemon wedges on the side.

Amount Per Serving

Calories 40   Calories from Fat 1   Total Calories From: Fat 3% Protein 6% Carb. 91%

Vitamin A 4%   Vitamin C 86%   Iron 1%

Grapefruit Ice

After a hot spicy meal, top off the evening with this refreshingly simple dessert, or serve between courses to cleanse the palate.

4 SERVINGS

2 tablespoons fructose

2 cups fresh grapefruit juice from ruby red grapefruit or other rose-fleshed grapefruits

pink grapefruit segments, for garnish

4 sprigs of mint, for garnish

1. Stir fructose into grapefruit juice to dissolve (save grapefruit shell). Turn into ice cream maker and freeze according to manufacturer's instructions, or place in freezer until slushy, then beat again before serving.

2. Serve in the grapefruit shell garnished with several grapefruit segments and a sprig of mint.

Amount Per Serving

Calories 76   Calories from Fat 1   Total Calories From: Fat 1% Protein 3% Carb. 96%

Vitamin A 11%   Vitamin C 76%   Iron 1%

Cantaloupe Sorbet

Sit back in a fancy wicker chair and enjoy your own taste of paradise!

4 SERVINGS

1 cantaloupe

2 tablespoons fructose

1 tablespoon fresh lemon juice

pinch of very finely grated lemon zest

1. Cut cantaloupe in half, remove seeds, cut pulp from rind, and cut cantaloupe into large chunks.

2. Combine cantaloupe, fructose, and lemon juice in blender or food processor and purée until smooth.

3. Add the lemon zest. Put into ice cream maker and freeze according to manufacturer's instructions, or place in freezer until slushy.

4. Sorbet may be served immediately but is a little firmer if transferred to a chilled storage container and placed in freezer for 30 minutes before serving. Store in freezer for up to a week; let soften for a few minutes before serving if too firm.

Amount Per Serving

Calories 82   Calories from Fat 3   Total Calories From: Fat 4% Protein 6% Carb. 90%

Vitamin A 86%   Vitamin C 97%   Iron 2%

Pineapple Supreme

Hot pineapple drizzled with honey and vinegar has a tart-sweet flavor that you'll love.

6 SERVINGS

¼ cup honey

2 tablespoons cider vinegar

1 tablespoon crystallized ginger, finely chopped

1 medium-size ripe pineapple, peeled and cored

fresh sprigs of basil, for garnish

1. In a small pan, combine honey, vinegar, and ginger. Stir over low heat until warm for about 3 minutes and set aside.

2. Cut pineapple crosswise into ½-inch thick slices or cut lengthwise into ½-inch thick wedges. Arrange pineapple pieces in a single layer in a shallow-rimmed baking pan and drizzle with honey mixture.

3. Broil about 4 inches below heat until pineapple is lightly browned (3 to 4 minutes). Using a wide spatula, transfer pineapple to a warm platter or plates. Spoon pan juices over pineapple and garnish with basil sprigs, if desired.

Amount Per Serving

Calories 217   Calories from Fat 12   Total Calories From: Fat 6% Protein 2% Carb. 92%

Vitamin A 1%   Vitamin C 78%   Iron 7%

Cantaloupe in Strawberry Purée

This dessert is the delightful result of having too many strawberries and cantaloupe on hand at the height of the season, when succulent, unblemished strawberries and cantaloupe are in abundance. This stunningly simple dessert is not to be missed. The look is beautiful, the taste divine.

4 SERVINGS

1½ cups strawberries, rinsed and drained

2½ tablespoons fructose

¼ cup cream sherry

1 cantaloupe, quartered, seeded, and rind removed

mint leaf, for garnish

1. Reserve 4 strawberries for garnish and blend the remaining strawberries in a blender or food processor until puréed.

2. Combine strawberry purée, fructose, and sherry in a 1-quart pan. Cook over medium-high heat, stirring, until fructose is dissolved and mixture is boiling. Boil for additional 25-30 seconds. Remove from heat and let cool. (At this stage you may cover and let stand for up to 1 hour.)

3. Thinly slice the cantaloupe. Spoon the strawberry purée onto individual dessert plates; arrange cantaloupe decoratively over sauce. Garnish with reserved strawberries and mint leaves.

Amount Per Serving

Calories 130   Calories from Fat 5   Total Calories From: Fat 5% Protein 6% Carb. 89%

Vitamin A 86%   Vitamin C 147%   Iron 3%

Tofu Cream Topping

Need something to add that last-minute flair to your fruit? Try this, and you'll love it.

6 SERVINGS

1 8-ounce package low-fat silken tofu

1 tablespoon fresh lemon juice

**2 tablespoons honey,
or substitute maple syrup, rice syrup,
or apple juice concentrate**

¼ teaspoon cardamom (optional)

Blend all ingredients thoroughly in a blender or food processor. This is great served over Vanilla Pudding with Berries (see page 232) or serve it with a bowl of fresh berries.

Amount Per Serving

Calories 45	Calories from Fat 12	Total Calories From: Fat 27% Protein 61% Carb. 12%
		Vitamin A 0% Vitamin C 0% Iron 30%

Raspberry-Banana Whip

There is no cream in this whip, but the flavor will have you fooled!

4 SERVINGS

2 very ripe large bananas

1 tablespoon fresh lemon juice

1 cup fresh raspberries

pinch of lemon zest, very finely grated

1. Peel bananas, remove fibers, and cut into chunks. Dip into lemon juice. Place on cookie sheet and put into freezer. Clean raspberries and place on cookie sheet. Freeze at least 2 hours.

2. Place frozen bananas and raspberries in a food processor or blender and whip until thick and creamy. Add lemon zest and whirl to blend. Serve immediately.

Amount Per Serving

Calories 76   Calories from Fat 4   Total Calories From: Fat 5% Protein 5% Carb. 90%

Vitamin A 2%   Vitamin C 24%   Iron 2%

Creamy Raspberry Pudding

This recipe uses agar, a tasteless sea vegetable rich in fiber, and kudzu, the root of the kudzu plant, which grows wild in the southern states of the U.S. Most of the kudzu you will find is imported from Japan, since there is no American company producing and marketing it. By using both agar and kudzu as thickeners, you get a smooth, creamy dessert.

8 SERVINGS

1 quart raspberry nectar*

2 cups fresh raspberries

⅓ cup agar flakes (see glossary)

1 tablespoon kudzu dissolved in ¼ cup water (see glossary)

2 tablespoons raspberry jam

1 teaspoon vanilla extract

fresh raspberries, for garnish

1. Put nectar and 1 cup fresh raspberries in a medium saucepan over medium heat. Sprinkle agar on top and bring to a boil. Lower heat and simmer for 10 minutes or until agar flakes are completely dissolved.

2. Add dissolved kudzu in water, stirring mixture constantly until smooth and clear. Remove from heat and add jam and vanilla extract. Stir again.

3. Pour into a 9 x 13-inch pan and let jell at room temperature for an hour. When jelled, pour the mixture into a blender and blend for a few seconds until smooth.

4. Pour into individual serving cups. Garnish with fresh raspberries on top and serve.

*Look for raspberry nectar in your health food store.

Amount Per Serving

Calories 51	Calories from Fat 5	Total Calories From: Fat 8% Protein 7% Carb. 85%
		Vitamin A 2% Vitamin C 38% Iron 3%

Vanilla Pudding with Berries

This creamy pudding is a great way to end a special meal. To make the dessert even tastier, serve it with Scrumptious Strawberry Sauce (see page 238) drizzled on the plate, and spoon berries over the top and around the pudding as decoration.

SERVINGS

1 cup nonfat vanilla soymilk

1 cup amasake (see glossary)

2 tablespoons agar flakes
(see glossary)

1 tablespoon kudzu,
dissolved in ¼ cup water
(see glossary)

2 tablespoons brown rice syrup

1 tablespoon vanilla extract

¼ teaspoon ground nutmeg

2 cups fresh berries, such as raspberries,
strawberries, or blueberries

1. Put soymilk and amasake into a medium-size saucepan over medium heat. Sprinkle agar on top. Simmer 10 minutes or until flakes have dissolved.

2. Add kudzu. Whisk until mixture thickens. Add syrup and stir again. Remove from heat.

3. Stir in vanilla extract. Let it set at room temperature for about an hour.

4. Once the pudding has set, put the mixture into the blender or food processor for a few seconds to create a creamy pudding texture.

5. Pour into individual serving cups and sprinkle a little nutmeg over each serving. Surround the pudding with fresh berries.

Amount Per Serving

Calories 5   Calories from Fat 0   Total Calories From: Fat 9% Protein 1% Carb. 90%

Vitamin A 0%   Vitamin C 0%   Iron 0%

Quick Rice Pudding

Served hot or cold, this healthy rice pudding will have you coming back for more.

4 SERVINGS

2½ cups cooked short-grain brown rice

1½ cup nonfat soymilk

1 medium Granny Smith apple, diced

⅓ cup brown sugar

⅓ cup raisins

⅓ cup dried apricots, chopped

½ teaspoon ground cinnamon

⅛ teaspoon ground ginger

½ teaspoon ground nutmeg, for garnish

½ fresh apple, thinly sliced, for garnish

1. Combine the cooked rice, soymilk, apple, sugar, raisins, apricots, cinnamon, and ginger in a medium saucepan. Cook over medium-low heat, stirring often, about 15 minutes or until the rice is thick and the fruit is tender. Remove from heat and let cool slightly before serving.

2. When ready to serve, spoon the rice pudding into bowls and garnish each serving with a sliver of apple.

Amount Per Serving

Calories 531   Calories from Fat 66   Total Calories From: Fat 13% Protein 7% Carb. 80%

Vitamin A 0%   Vitamin C 1%   Iron 11%

Chocolate Soufflé

Soufflés have the reputation of being difficult to make. In fact, this soufflé is nothing more than an airy, chocolatey baked pudding that is fluffed up high with beaten egg whites. The only real challenge is making sure that you are ready when the soufflé is. Once removed from the oven, it waits for no one.

4 SERVINGS

5 egg whites

¼ teaspoon sea salt
or salt substitute

¼ teaspoon cream of tartar

⅔ cup fructose

3 ounces Ghirardelli semi-sweet
chocolate chips

Tofu Cream Topping (optional)

1. Preheat oven to 425° F. Beat egg whites until foamy. Sprinkle salt and cream of tartar over the egg whites and beat until stiff, but not dry. Gradually beat in fructose.

2. Melt chocolate chips and fold into the stiffened egg whites. Pour the mixture into an ungreased 1-quart soufflé dish or four small individual soufflé dishes. Bake 20 to 25 minutes for the 1-quart soufflé dish or 15-20 minutes for the small soufflé dishes, or until well puffed and browned.

3. Serve immediately with a dollop of Tofu Cream Topping (see page 229), if desired.

Amount Per Serving

Calories 291	Calories from Fat 68	Total Calories From: Fat 24% Protein 7% Carb. 69%
Vitamin A 0%	Vitamin C 0%	Iron 3%

Winter Fruit Compote

Dried fruit was traditionally served in winter when fresh fruit was unavailable. However, we eat it just because it tastes great!

4 SERVINGS

1 cup fresh orange juice

¼ cup fresh lemon juice

½ cup water

1 cinnamon stick

6 cloves

2 ¼-inch slices peeled fresh ginger

2 pears, peeled, cored,
and cut into 8 sections each

1 Granny Smith apple, peeled, cored,
and cut into 8 sections

½ cup dried cherries

½ cup dried apricots, diced

¼ cup raisins

1. In a 2-quart saucepan, combine juices, water, cinnamon stick, cloves, and ginger. Bring mixture to a boil, reduce heat to low, and simmer 12 minutes.

2. Add pears, apple, cherries, apricots, and raisins to saucepan. Simmer until fruit is tender, about 16 minutes.

3. Remove fruit from poaching liquid. Strain the liquid and return to cleaned saucepan. Boil the liquid until it is reduced and syrupy, 6 to 8 minutes. Pour the syrup over the fruit. Serve warm or chilled.

Amount Per Serving

Calories 245   Calories from Fat 7   Total Calories From: Fat 3% Protein 4% Carb. 93%

Vitamin A 41%   Vitamin C 76%   Iron 10%

Silken Tofu in Ginger Sauce

Toi, a friend from Thailand, first made this recipe while visiting our home. This dish, I am told, is a very common dessert in Thailand. The recipe below is my variation of this traditional dish.

8 SERVINGS

1 pound nonfat silken tofu

3 cups water

4 tablespoons rice syrup

8 slices of ginger root,
sliced the size of a silver dollar

1. Bring 3 cups of water to boil in a saucepan. Add the ginger root and rice syrup. Lower heat and simmer for 20 minutes.

2. Slice the tofu thinly and add enough water to cover. Heat to a boil. Remove from stove and drain the water. Divide the tofu into four equal servings and put into serving bowls.

3. Pour the hot ginger root rice syrup sauce over the tofu and serve.

Amount Per Serving

Calories 45   Calories from Fat 12   Total Calories From: Fat 27% Protein 61% Carb. 12%

Vitamin A 0%   Vitamin C 0%   Iron 30%

Strawberries with Gingered Vanilla Sauce

Fruit sauces as dips, toppings, or mixed into fruit salad make this simple dish one you'll come back to time and time again.

2 SERVINGS

1 pound strawberries with stems, rinsed and drained

¾ cup nonfat silken tofu

2 very ripe bananas, sliced

½ teaspoon vanilla extract

¼ teaspoon fresh ginger root, finely shredded

1. In a blender or food processor, blend the tofu, banana, vanilla, and ginger root into a smooth sauce.

2. Drizzle a design on the serving plate with the sauce. Arrange berries on the plate.

3. Offer the remaining sauce on the side.

Amount Per Serving

Calories 167   Calories from Fat 16   Total Calories From: Fat 10% Protein 12% Carb. 78%

Vitamin A 2%   Vitamin C 216%   Iron 5%

Scrumptious Strawberry Sauce

For a quick and easy sauce for that platter of fruit, this is just the ticket. Your guests will love it!

4 SERVINGS

1 pint fresh strawberries, washed and trimmed

1 tablespoon fresh orange juice

½ teaspoon lemon juice

1 banana

1. Place all but 6 strawberries, juices, and banana in blender and blend until smooth.

2. Pour sauce into serving dish and add fruit, or make a design on your plate with the sauce and arrange the fresh fruit attractively. Use remaining strawberries for garnish. Will keep several days in the refrigerator.

Amount Per Serving

Calories 26   Calories from Fat 2   Total Calories From: Fat 10% Protein 7% Carb. 83%

Vitamin A 0%   Vitamin C 71%   Iron 2%

Beverages

▼

The best beverage to drink requires little preparation and is nearly impossible to consume in excess — water. In fact, most people fail to drink as much of this vital liquid as health experts recommend, a minimum of eight glasses a day. But sometimes you just want something with more flavor or texture. These recipes blend the goodness of fresh fruits and other wholesome ingredients into luscious beverages. Add one to a meal, or sip one as a cool and refreshing treat. These drinks are low in fat and high in carbohydrates, nutrients, and taste. And you can create your own special concoctions by varying the fruit and other ingredients according to what's in season … or in the refrigerator.

Try Water

Chilled water with a slice of lemon or lime makes a tasty thirst-quencher that's good for you, too. Health experts say adults should drink at least eight glasses of water a day.

Green Tea

Green tea can be served the traditional way, hot, or try it poured over ice with lemon and a sprig of mint.

1 SERVING

1 teaspoon green tea or 1 green tea bag

8 ounces boiling water

fruit concentrate (optional)

To make green tea, bring water to a boil and pour over tea. Let tea steep for 3 minutes. If using a tea bag, press the bag before removing to enhance the flavor.

In the summer months when we're looking for a refreshing cool drink, I often freeze the green tea in my ice cube tray, transferring the cubes to resealable bags for later use in my iced tea, thereby avoiding dilution of the tea when I want it iced. Add a slice of lemon, a sprig of mint, or a teaspoon of fruit concentrate to vary the taste.

Amount Per Serving

Calories 0   Calories from Fat 0   Total Calories From: Fat 0% Protein 0% Carb. 0%

Vitamin A 0%   Vitamin C 0%   Iron 0%

Ginger Tea

This is an extra-special treat on a cold winter night.

2 SERVINGS

1 2-inch piece ginger root, thinly sliced

2 cups boiling water

2 slices lemon

2 teaspoons honey or maple syrup, to taste (optional)

1. Place the ginger root in a pot with the water and simmer 15-20 minutes.

2. Strain, and pour the simmered liquid into cups. Add a squeeze of fresh lemon and stir in honey or maple syrup to taste if you wish a sweeter taste.

Amount Per Serving

Calories 49   Calories from Fat 2   Total Calories From: Fat 3% Protein 5% Carb. 92%

Vitamin A 0%   Vitamin C 51%   Iron 2%

Citrus Water

This is a great thirst-quencher anytime, but especially with summer meals. Keep a pitcher of citrus water in the refrigerator. Vary it by adding all lemon, all lime, or all orange slices.

8 SERVINGS

2 quarts water

¼ lemon, thinly sliced

¼ orange, thinly sliced

¼ lime, thinly sliced

Put water into a pitcher and add the lemon, orange, and lime slices. Let it set ½ hour or longer. Refrigerate or drink at room temperature.

Amount Per Serving

Calories 4   Calories from Fat 0   Total Calories From: Fat 3% Protein 7% Carb. 90%

Vitamin A 0%   Vitamin C 6%   Iron 0%

Citrus Delight

I enjoyed this drink for the first time a year ago while visiting a friend in Florida. It was hot and humid outside. We picked fresh oranges and grapefruit from my friend's trees, went into the house and made this cool, refreshing drink. It's also good with a little fresh ginger root juice added.

4 SERVINGS

4 medium pink grapefruits

4 medium oranges

1 small lemon

1 small lime

fresh basil, finely chopped, for garnish

1. Halve and squeeze the grapefruits, oranges, lemon, and lime. Strain the juices into a bowl, discarding the pulp and seeds, or process in your juicer.

2. Pour the citrus delight into 4 tall ice-filled glasses, garnish with fresh basil, and serve.

Amount Per Serving

Calories 166   Calories from Fat 0   Total Calories From: Fat 3% Protein 7% Carb. 90%

Vitamin A 18%   Vitamin C 294%   Iron 4%

Grape Juice Sangria

For a hot summer day, freeze sparkling water in your ice cube trays, and replace the crushed ice in this drink with sparkling crushed ice. It's a great pick-me-upper!

4 SERVINGS

2 cups fresh strawberries

2 oranges

1 lime

1 Jonathan apple (or other apple of choice), core removed and cut into ¼-inch slices

1½ cups white grape juice

crushed ice

1. Wash all the fruit. Hull and halve the strawberries.

2. Juice the oranges and lime. Place the apple and strawberries in a pitcher, pour in the orange, lime, and grape juice, and stir.

3. Refrigerate the sangria for at least 2 hours. To serve, pour the sangria into 4 ice-filled glasses and divide the fruit among them.

Amount Per Serving

Calories 91   Calories from Fat 5   Total Calories From: Fat 4% Protein 6% Carb. 90%

Vitamin A 2%   Vitamin C 121%   Iron 3%

Sparkling Fruit Juice

This is even better if you freshly squeeze the juice and save a slice of the fruit to decorate the top of the glass.

4 SERVINGS

2 cups sparkling water

2 cups orange juice, or other juice of your choice

Combine the sparkling water with the fruit juice and serve chilled or at room temperature.

Amount Per Serving

Calories 59   Calories from Fat 3   Total Calories From: Fat 5% Protein 7% Carb. 88%

Vitamin A 2%   Vitamin C 71%   Iron 1%

Banana Milk

For that extra-healthy, extra-simple treat, try this one.

2 SERVINGS

1 banana, cut into large chunks

2 cups nonfat soymilk

2 teaspoons vanilla extract

Blend the banana, soymilk, and vanilla extract in your blender or food processor and serve.

Amount Per Serving

Calories 128   Calories from Fat 5   Total Calories From: Fat 4% Protein 4% Carb. 92%

Vitamin A 2%   Vitamin C 17%   Iron 2%

Apricot Tofu Breakfast

This is a very filling breakfast starter. I like to substitute fresh apricots for the dried when they are in season.

1 SERVING

1 8-ounce package soft or silken tofu

6 dried organic apricots

¼ cup orange juice

juice of ½ lemon

2 tablespoons oat or bran flakes

Combine all ingredients in a blender and blend until thick and fairly smooth. The oat or bran flakes give this drink body. It will thicken more if you let it stand for five minutes before you drink it.

Amount Per Serving

Calories 310   Calories from Fat 106   Total Calories From: Fat 34% Protein 28% Carb. 38%

Vitamin A 123%   Vitamin C 38%   Iron 74%

Tofu-Berry Shake

This shake is a perfect way to get a running start on the day's activities. Strawberries, blueberries, and raspberries are my favorite fruits. I grow my own wild strawberries and they are a lot smaller than the ones you find in your supermarket, but oooh, how sweet and delicious they are!

2 SERVINGS

½ cup nonfat silken tofu

1 cup either strawberries, blueberries, or raspberries, or any combination

½ cup soymilk

juice from half a lime

6 ice cubes

½ banana

Combine all ingredients in a blender or food processor and blend until smooth.

Amount Per Serving

Calories 130   Calories from Fat 8   Total Calories From: Fat 6% Protein 24% Carb. 70%

Vitamin A 3%   Vitamin C 53%   Iron 4%

Spicy Yam Shake

Use cooked sweet potatoes or cooked acorn squash for variety. It's a meal in a glass!

1 SERVING

½ cup yam, cooked and well-chilled

1 ounce low-fat silken tofu

1 tablespoon honey

½ cup nonfat soymilk

pinch of ground ginger

pinch of pumpkin pie spice

1. Combine the first 3 ingredients in a blender and blend for 10 seconds. Add the soymilk and spices and blend for another 5 seconds.

2. Pour the shake into a tall glass and serve.

Amount Per Serving

Calories 129   Calories from Fat 13   Total Calories From: Fat 10% Protein 9% Carb. 81%

Vitamin A 110%   Vitamin C 25%   Iron 12%

Raspberry-Rice Shake

I first made this drink for a Japanese student I was hosting. She was accustomed to eating rice for breakfast, so we mixed up this blend to her delight! We vary the shake depending on what fruit we have available in the house. The combinations are endless.

2 SERVINGS

½ cup brown rice, cooked and cooled

1 ripe banana, peeled and cut into chunks

1 cup unsweetened frozen raspberries

¼ cup low-fat silken tofu

¾ cup nonfat soymilk

2 teaspoons honey

1. Place the rice in a food processor or blender and blend until puréed, scraping down the sides of the container with a rubber spatula. Add the banana and blend for another 30 seconds, or until the mixture is as smooth as possible. Add the raspberries, tofu, soymilk, and honey, and blend for another 15 seconds.

2. Divide the shake between 2 glasses and serve.

Amount Per Serving

Calories 285   Calories from Fat 18   Total Calories From: Fat 6% Protein 7% Carb. 87%

Vitamin A 3%   Vitamin C 34%   Iron 7%

Breakfast Berry Shake

If you have fruit nectar on hand, it makes a great substitute for the soymilk or rice milk and adds a new dimension to this tasty shake.

4 SERVINGS

5 ounces firm, low-fat silken tofu

½ cup frozen strawberries (organic unsweetened, if available)

8 ounces vanilla-flavored nonfat soymilk or rice milk

8 ounces all-fruit premium-blend juice

2 bananas

fresh fruit, for garnish (optional)

4 mint sprigs, for garnish (optional)

Mix all ingredients in a blender and purée until smooth and creamy. Add additional milk to reach desired consistency. Garnish with fresh fruit or mint sprigs, if desired.

Amount Per Serving

Calories 310   Calories from Fat 106   Total Calories From: Fat 34% Protein 28% Carb. 38%

Vitamin A 123%   Vitamin C 38%   Iron 74%

Glossary

Most of the recipes in this book use familiar ingredients that you'll find at your local supermarket. There are, however, special ingredients in some of the recipes that may be new to you. You'll find that using these new ingredients in your cooking will make your dishes more interesting and help you to become a more creative cook. While most of these ingredients can be found in larger supermarkets, health food stores, and Asian markets, some of them may be more difficult to locate. Consult the resources section at the end of the book for the addresses of mail order companies that carry uncommon or hard-to-find ingredients.

Agar, a sea vegetable, is a natural jelling agent that can be used in place of animal gelatin. When added to liquids at room temperature, agar acts as a thickener, whereas gelatin must be added to hot water to dissolve the crystals, and then the mixture must be chilled for thickening or jelling to occur. One-quarter cup of agar jels a quart of liquid. Agar is sold in bars or flakes, but flakes are easier to measure. Look for agar in your natural food store.

Amasake is a traditional Japanese liquid used as a sweetening agent. It is made by fermenting sweet brown rice into a thick, sweet liquid. You will find it either in an aseptic package on the shelf or in the refrigerated section of your natural food store.

Balsamic vinegar is an aromatic Italian vinegar made from grapes. It has a sweeter flavor than most vinegars.

Black bean sauce is a thick, salty sauce made from fermented yellow soybeans, flour, and salt. Brown bean sauce can be purchased from your Asian market and comes packed in cans, jars, or plastic packages. Refrigerate, tightly covered, after opening.

Dark soy sauce can be substituted for black bean sauce.

Bouquet garni, or herb bouquet as it is sometimes called, refers to a combination of parsley, thyme, and bay leaf. It is used most often for flavoring soups, stews, sauces, and braised vegetables. A small bouquet should contain 2 parsley sprigs, ⅓ of a bay leaf, and 1 sprig of thyme.

Couscous is a North African grain that is actually a quick-cooking form of wheat. It's made from the same type of wheat as pasta, and cooks up to resemble very tiny pearled versions of pasta.

Daikon is a giant white radish that is sold in Asian markets. It can be cooked, sliced and eaten raw in salads, or grated and used as a garnish.

Fish sauce is a salty, pale brown liquid used widely in Thai cooking. It is made from fermented small fish or shrimp. The fish are salted and fermented in jars and then the liquid is collected. It adds salt to many dishes and is essential for authentic Thai flavors. Fish sauce is available in Asian food stores.

Galangal, a relative of the ginger root, is pale yellow and has a unique, delicate flavor, and can be obtained as a root knob or in dried or powdered form from Asian food stores. Fresh young ginger root is an adequate substitute for galangal, but does not properly replace its unique flavor. In Indonesia, galangal is called laos.

Hoisin sauce is a thick, sweet, reddish-brown sauce usually made from soybeans, vinegar, chilies, spices, and garlic and used in cooking and as a table condiment in China. You will find this in your Asian market, or order by mail (see the Resources section in the back of this book).

Kombu, also known as kelp, is a dark green sea vegetable sold in thick strips. It contains glutamic acid, which acts as a tenderizer when added to cooking beans. As with other sea vegetables, kombu is mineral-rich. Store kombu in a sealed container in a cool, dark place, where it will keep indefinitely.

Kudzu is a white starch made from the root of the wild kudzu plant. In this country, the plant densely populates the southern states. It is used in making soups, sauces, desserts, and medicinal beverages. You will find it in any well-stocked health food store.

Mirin is sake, or Japanese rice wine, that has been sweetened. It gives food sweetness and a glaze. You can combine 1 tablespoon sake and 1 teaspoon sugar for mirin.

Miso is fermented soybean paste that usually also contains a grain (barley or rice). There are many different kinds of miso. Some are salty, some are sweet. Hatcho-miso is dark in color and has a wonderful flavor. White miso is sweet and is used for some salad dressings. Use as a condiment to add a deep, rich, salty flavor to soups and other dishes. The type of miso you use for miso soup is mostly a matter of personal taste. Do not boil or reheat miso, as this destroys the enzymes that are so beneficial for your health.

Miso is usually sold in transparent plastic packages, and keeps well in an airtight container or plastic bag in the refrigerator.

Nutritional yeast is a nutrient-rich inactive yeast. It doesn't have any leavening power, but rather adds nutrition and a "cheesy" flavor to dishes. It comes in a powder or flake form. Look for it in your health food store or order by mail (see the Resources section at the back of this book).

Seitan is a wheat gluten cooked in tamari soy sauce, kelp, and water, and is used as a meat substitute in cooking. You will find it in the refrigerated section of your health food store.

Tamarind juice comes from the fruit of the tamarind tree. The fruit is eaten green, and the brown pulp is used for cooking. Tamarind juice adds a sharp, sour flavor to your dishes without the tartness of lemon. It can be prepared at home or bought in bottles at Asian food markets. To make tamarind juice yourself, combine 1 tablespoon of tamarind paste with ½ cup of hot water and stir. Commercial tamarind sauce can be used as a substitute for tamarind juice by diluting a small amount of the sauce with water. Lemon or lime can also be used as a substitute in a pinch, but the delicate flavor will be lost.

Tempeh is a rich-tasting, fermented soybean cake. This is a staple in Indonesian cooking and makes a wonderful meat substitute in chili or on the grill.

Textured vegetable protein is a food product made from soybeans that is used as a meat substitute. It is produced from soy flour after the soybean oil has been extracted, then cooked under pressure, extruded, and dried.

Wakame is a type of seaweed, bright green in color, with a delicate texture. It is most commonly used in miso soup, but can also be added to pickled cucumbers and other vegetables. Wakame is sold dried and already trimmed and cut in plastic packages, or in a long, dried strip that you have to cut yourself. Once opened, store it in an airtight container or plastic bag in the refrigerator.

RESOURCES

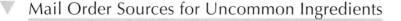

Mail Order Sources for Uncommon Ingredients

If you can't locate some of the ingredients used in this book, you can find everything you need through the sources listed below. Call and request a catalog, and you will be amazed at the bounty available.

Natural Lifestyle
16 Lookout Drive
Asheville, NC 28804-3330
Web site: www.natural-lifestyle.com
Telephone: (800) 752-2775
Excellent one-stop shopping for a wide range of soy products
and personal health care products.

Penzeys Spices
P. O. Box 933
W19362 Apollo Drive
Muskego, WI 53150
Web site: www.penzeys.com
Telephone: (800) 741-7787
Fax: (262) 679-7878
Great selection of dried herbs and spices with a
fascinating catalog full of tips on use and storage.

Dixie USA, Inc.
P.O. Box 55549
Houston, TX 77255
Web site: www.dixieusa.com/DDC.html
Telephone: (713) 688-4993
Fax: (800) 688-2507
A great source for soy products, cereals, dairy substitutes,
meatless entrée mixes, flours, and meat substitute mixes,
as well as cookbooks, kitchenware, and condiments.

Adriana's Caravan
409 Vanderbilt Street
Brooklyn, NY 11218
Telephone: (800) 316-0820
Fax: (718) 436-8565
A good source of ethnic condiments and ingredients,
such as Thai curry paste, fish sauce, tamarind sauce, and rice papers.

▼ Internet Resources and Web Sites
for Prostate Cancer Information

www.prostatepointers.org/prostate/edu-pip/glossary.html
Lists many sources of information on prostate cancer available on the Internet.

www.prostatepointers.org/prostate/pcsup.html
Telephone numbers for support groups across the country and around the world.

www.prostatepointers.org/calendar/index
Lists events of interest to prostate cancer patients.

www.webmd.com
Health news and information, a physician directory, and condition-specific
support groups.

www.prostatepointers.org/prostate/ed-pip/acronyms

Acronyms and abbreviations of interest to prostate cancer patients.

www.prostatepointers.org/prostate/

A site maintained by Gary Huckabay, lists a number of sources of information about the prostate and prostate cancer.

www.prostatepointers.org/pcan/

Prostate Cancer Action Network (PCAN)— A dedicated coalition of support organizations, patients, and their loved ones who actively and responsibly engage the issues, institutions, and individuals that impact the cure, care, and treatment of prostate cancer patients and survivors.

www.prostatepointers.org/prostate/resource

A prostate cancer resource list of useful information.

www.capcure.org/

CaP CURE, Association for the Cure of Cancer of the Prostate—Source of prostate cancer information including current research and clinical trials.

www.oncology.com

Source of information about cancer, including prostate cancer.

www.prostatepointers.org/information

List of useful sources of information about prostate cancer.

www.prostatepointers.org/strum/

Prostate Cancer Research Institute (PCRI)—A nonprofit educational and research center for prostate cancer.

www.prostatepointer.org/circle/

Called *The Circle*, this is a mailing list and associated website offering support for men with prostate cancer and their wives, families, and friends.

www.prostatepointers.org/seedpods/

A mailing list offering information and support for people interested in brachytherapy for prostate cancer.

www.intellihealth.com

IntelliHealth offers comprehensive medical information from Johns Hopkins Hospital.

www.mayohealth.org

Mayo Clinic Health Oasis

Includes a prescription drug index and a medical encyclopedia.

www.nlm.nih.gov/medlineplus

MedlinePlus—Provides a consumer version of the National Library of Medicine's resources for health professionals.

www.healthfinder.gov

Gives information from the Department of Health and Human Services. Healthfinder links to government agency health sites, online publications, and medical dictionaries.

www.medscape.com

Medscape—Original peer-reviewed reports and journal articles organized by medical specialty, designed for doctors.

www.americasdoctor.com

AmericasDoctor.com has chats and question-and-answer sessions with doctors.

www.fhcrc.org

Fred Hutchinson Cancer Research Center—World-renowned cancer research center. This website serves patients and the general public, as well as researchers.

www.oncolink.upenn.edu

Diverse site with huge article database on cancer.

www.centerwatch.com

Offers more than 40,000 clinical trials actively recruiting patients; includes research summaries.

www.cancer.org

American Cancer Society—Prevention strategies and news on lifestyle issues from the American Cancer Society.

www.cancernet.nci.nih.gov

National Cancer Institute (NCI), National Institutes of Health (NIH)

Up-to-date information on treatments and trials.

www.quackwatch.com

Attacks pseudoscience. Big list of quack sites.

REFERENCES

▼

Ahmad, N, et al: *Green tea constituent epigallocatechin-3-gallate and induction of apoptosis and cell cycle arrest in human carcinoma cells.* Journal of the National Cancer Institute. Vol. 89 (24), pp. 1881–1887, 12/17/97

Araki, H, et al: *High-risk group for benign prostatic hyperplasia.* The Prostate. Vol. 4, pp. 253–264, 1983

Chan, JM, et al: *What causes prostate cancer? A brief summary of the epidemiology.* Seminars in Cancer Biology. Vol. 8, pp. 263–273, Article #sc980075, 1998

Chyou, PH, et al: *A prospective study of alcohol, diet, and other lifestyle factors in relation to obstructive uropathy.* The Prostate. Vol. 22, pp. 253–264, 1993

Dorgan, JF, et al: *Effects of dietary fat and fiber on plasma and urine androgens and estrogens in men: a controlled feeding study.* American Journal of Clinical Nutrition. Vol. 54 (6), pp. 1093–1100, 4/17/91

Elstner, E, et al: *Novel 20-epi-vitamin D3 analog combined with 9-cis-retinoic acid markedly inhibits colony growth of prostate cancer cells.* The Prostate. Vol. 40, pp. 141–149, 1999

Fangliu, G: *Changes in the prevalence of benign prostatic hyperplasia in China.* Chinese Medical Journal. Vol. 110 (3), pp. 163–166, 1997

Fleshner, NE, Klotz, LH: *Diet, androgens, oxidative stress, and prostate cancer susceptibility.* Cancer Metastasis Review. Vol. 17, pp. 325–330, 1999

Folkman J: *What is the evidence that tumors are angiogenesis dependent?* Journal of the National Cancer Institute. Vol. 82 (1), pp. 4–6, 11/29/89

Gann, PH, et al: *Lower prostate cancer risk in men with elevated plasma lycopene levels.* Cancer Research. Vol. 59 (6), pp. 1225–1230, 3/15/99

Giovannucci, E, Ascherio, A, Rimm, EB, Stampfer, MJ, Colditz, GA, Willett, WC: *Intake of carotenoids and retinal in relation to risk of prostate cancer.* Journal of the National Cancer Institute. Vol. 87 (23), pp. 1767–1776, 12/06/95

Giovannucci, E, et al: *A prospective study of dietary fat and risk of prostate cancer.* Journal of the National Cancer Institute. Vol. 85 (19), pp. 1571–1579, 10/06/93

Herbert, JR, et al: *Nutritional and socioeconomic factors in relation to prostate cancer mortality, a cross-national study.* Journal of the National Cancer Institute. Vol. 90 (21), pp. 1637–1645, 11/04/98

Hisatake, J, et al: *5, 5-trans-16-ene-Vitamin D3: A new class of potent inhibitors of proliferation of prostate, breast, and myeloid leukemic cells.* Cancer Research. Vol. 59, pp. 4023–4029, 8/15/99

Howie, BJ, Shultz, TD: *Dietary and hormonal interrelationships among vegetarian Seventh-Day Adventists and nonvegetarian men.* American Journal of Clinical Nutrition. Vol. 42, pp. 127–134, 7/85

Kobayashi, M, et al: *Serum n-3 fatty acids, fish consumption and cancer mortality in six Japanese populations in Japan and Brazil.* Japan Journal of Cancer Research. Vol. 90, pp. 914–921, 9/99

Krill, D, et al: *Differential effects of vitamin D on normal human prostate epithelial and stromal cells in primary culture.* Urology. Vol. 54 (1), pp. 171–177, 2/08/99

Kristal, AR, et al: *Vitamin and mineral supplement use is associated with reduced risk of prostate cancer.* Cancer Epidemiology, Biomarkers & Prevention. Vol. 8, pp. 887–892, 10/99

Lagiou, P, et al: *Diet and benign prostatic hyperplasia: a study in Greece.* Urology. Vol. 54 (2), pp. 284–290, 1999

Lee, CT, Fair, WR: *The role of dietary manipulation in biochemical recurrence of prostate cancer after radical prostatectomy.* Seminars in Urologic Oncology. Vol. 17 (3), pp. 154–163, 8/99

Malter, M, Schriever, G, Eilber, U: *Natural killer cells, vitamins, and other blood components of vegetarian and omnivorous men.* Nutrition and Cancer. Vol. 12, pp. 271–278, 1989

Moyad, MA: *Soy, disease prevention, and prostate cancer.* Seminars in Urologic Oncology. Vol. 17 (2), pp. 97–102, 5/99

Nagasawa, H, Mitamura, T, Skaamoto, S, Yamamoto, K: *Effects of lycopene on spontaneous mammary tumor development in SHN virgin mice.* Anticancer Research. Vol.15 (4), pp. 1173–1178, 1995

Nelson, MA, et al: *Selenium and prostate cancer prevention.* Seminars in Urologic Oncology. Vol. 17 (2), pp. 91–96, 5/99

Niukian, K, et al: *Effects of onion extract on the development of hamster buccal pouch carcinomas as expressed in tumor burden.* Nutrition and Cancer. Vol. 9 (2&3), pp. 171–176, 1987

Pienta, KJ, et al: *Inhibition of spontaneous metastasis in a rat prostate cancer model by oral administration of modified citrus pectin.* Journal of the National Cancer Institute. Vol. 87 (5) pp., 348–353, 3/01/95

Pinto, JT, et al: *Effects of garlic thioallyl derivatives on growth, glutathione concentration, and polyamine formation of human prostate carcinoma cells in cultures.* American Journal of Clinical Nutrition. Vol. 66, pp. 398–405, 5/15/97

Pollard, M: *Prevention of prostate-related cancers in Lobund-Wistar rats.* The Prostate. Vol. 39, pp. 305–309, 1999

Rao, AV, Fleshner, N, Agarwal, S: *Serum and tissue lycopene and biomarkers of oxidation in prostate cancer patients: a case control study.* Nutrition and Cancer. Vol. 33 (2), pp. 150–164, 1999

Ripple, MO, et al: *Pro-oxidant-antioxidant shift induced by androgen treatment of human prostate carcinoma cells.* Journal of the National Cancer Institute. Vol. 89 (1), pp. 40–48, 1/01/97

Ross, RK, Henderson, BE: *Do diet and androgens alter prostate cancer risk via a common etiologic pathway?* Journal of the National Cancer Institute. Vol. 86 (4), pp. 252–254, 2/16/94

Shklar, G, et al: *Tumor necrosis factor in experimental cancer regression with alphatocopherol, beta-carotene, canthaxanthin and algae extract.* European Journal of Cancer and Clinical Oncology. Vol. 24 (5), pp. 839–850, 11/98

Talbott, MC, et al: *Pyridoxine supplementation: effect on lymphocyte responses in elderly persons.* American Journal of Clinical Nutrition. Vol. 46, pp. 659–664, 1/87

Thomas, JA: *Diet, micronutrients, and the prostate gland.* Nutrition Review. Vol. 57 (4), pp. 95–103, 4/99

West, DW, et al: *Adult dietary intake and prostate cancer risk in Utah: a case-control study with special emphasis on aggressive tumors.* Cancer Causes and Control. Vol. 2, pp. 85–94, 1991

Whittemore, AS, et al: *Prostate cancer in relation to diet, physical activity, and body size in blacks, whites, and Asians in the United States and Canada.* Journal of the National Cancer Institute. Vol. 87 (9), pp. 652–660, 5/03/95

Whittemore, AS, et al: *Low-grade, latent prostate cancer volume: predictor of clinical cancer incidence?* Journal of the National Cancer Institute. Vol. 83 (17), pp. 1231–1235, 9/04/91

Willett, WC, et al: *Diet and cancer: an overview.* New England Journal of Medicine. Vol. 310 (11), pp. 697–702, 3/15/84

Zhang, Y, Talalay, P, Cho, CG, Posner, GH: *A major inducer of anticarcinogenic protective enzymes from broccoli: Isolation and elucidation of structure.* Proceedings of the National Academy of Science, U.S.A. Vol. 89 (6), pp. 2399–2403, 3/92

Zhou, JR, et al: *Soybean phytochemicals inhibit the growth of transplantable human prostate carcinoma and tumor angiogenesis in mice.* Journals of Nutrition. Vol. 129 (9), pp. 1628–1635, 6/08/99

Index

▼